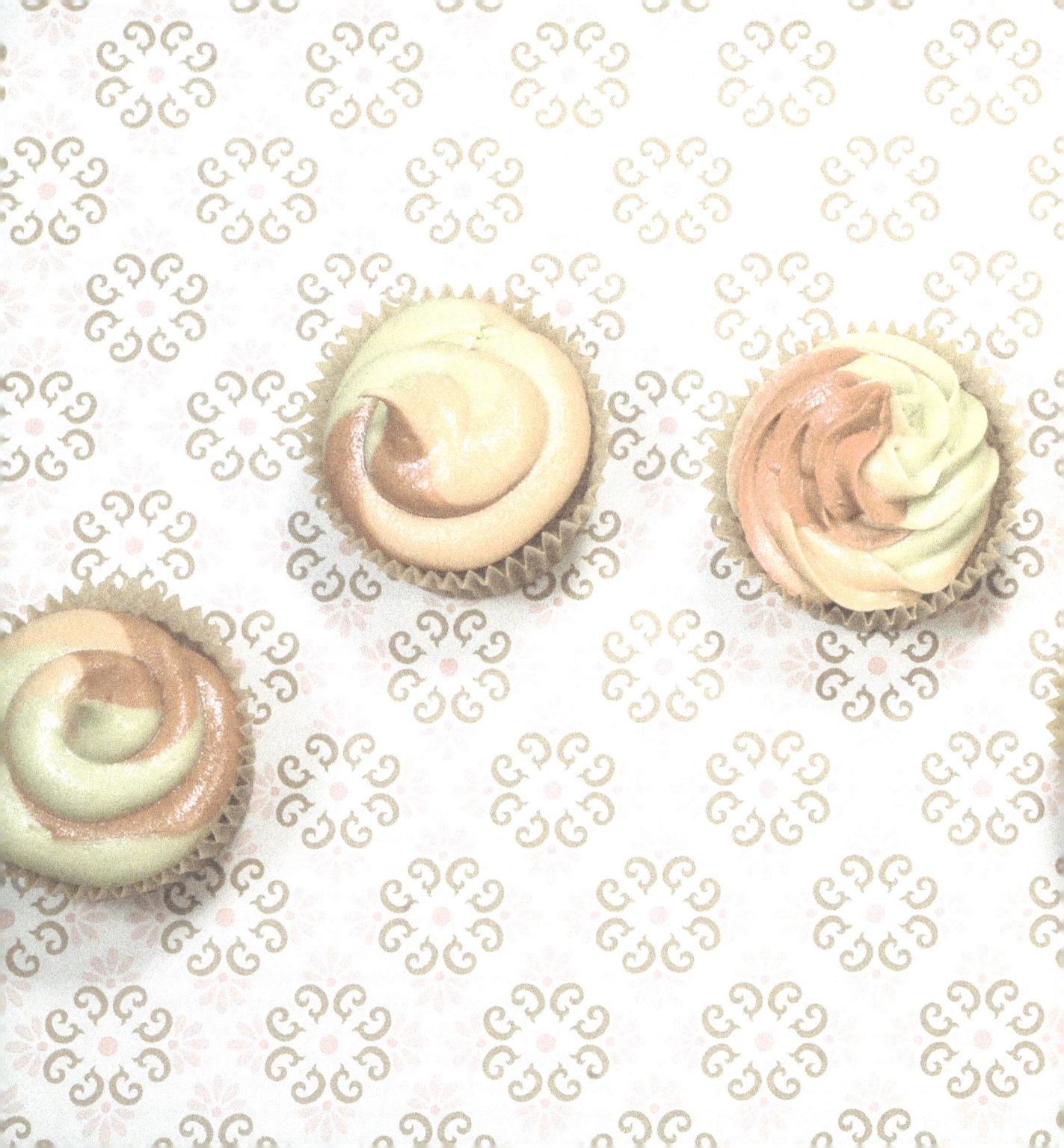

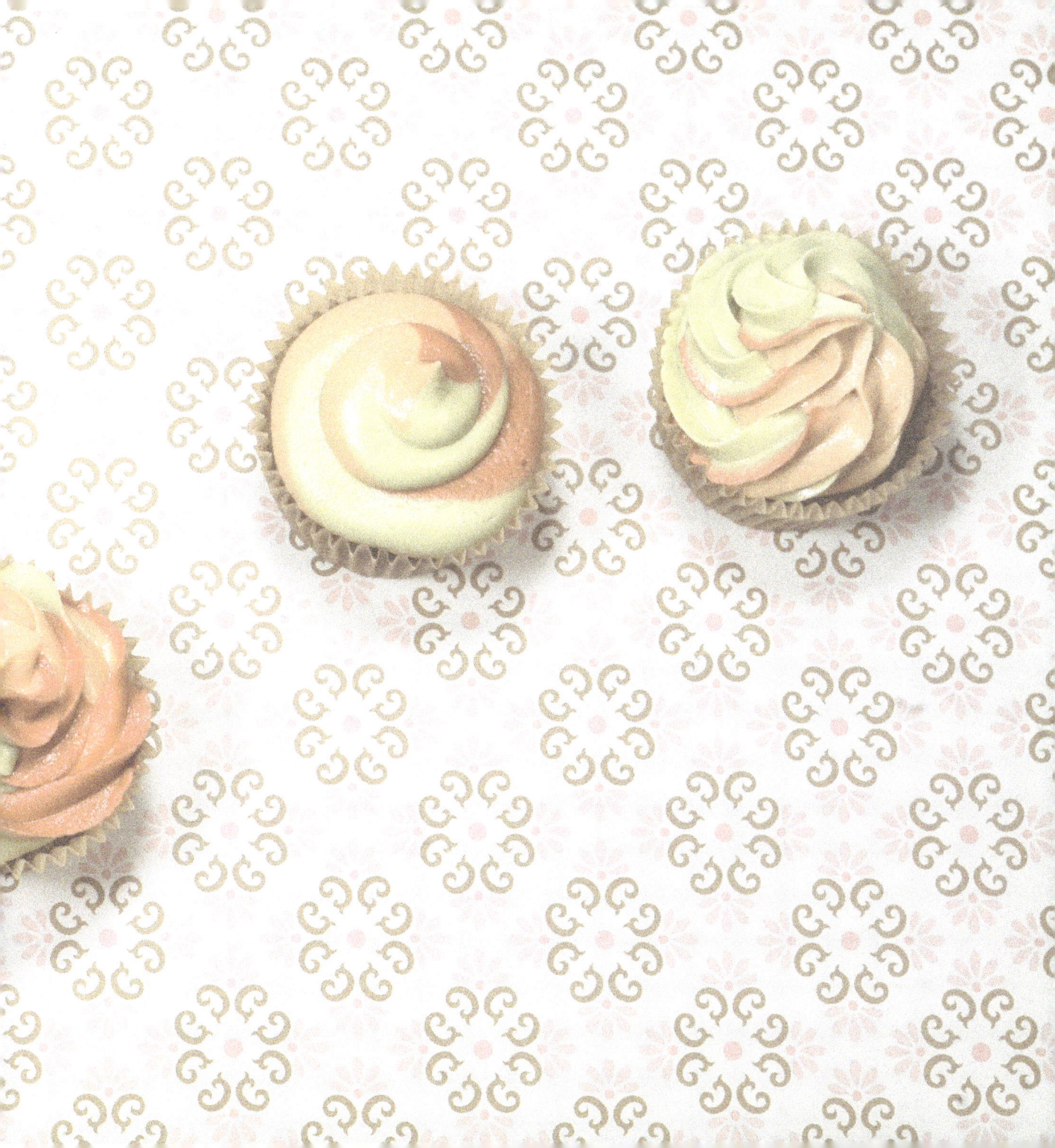

Sweets & Treats

Delicious recipes for those with food allergies and special diets.

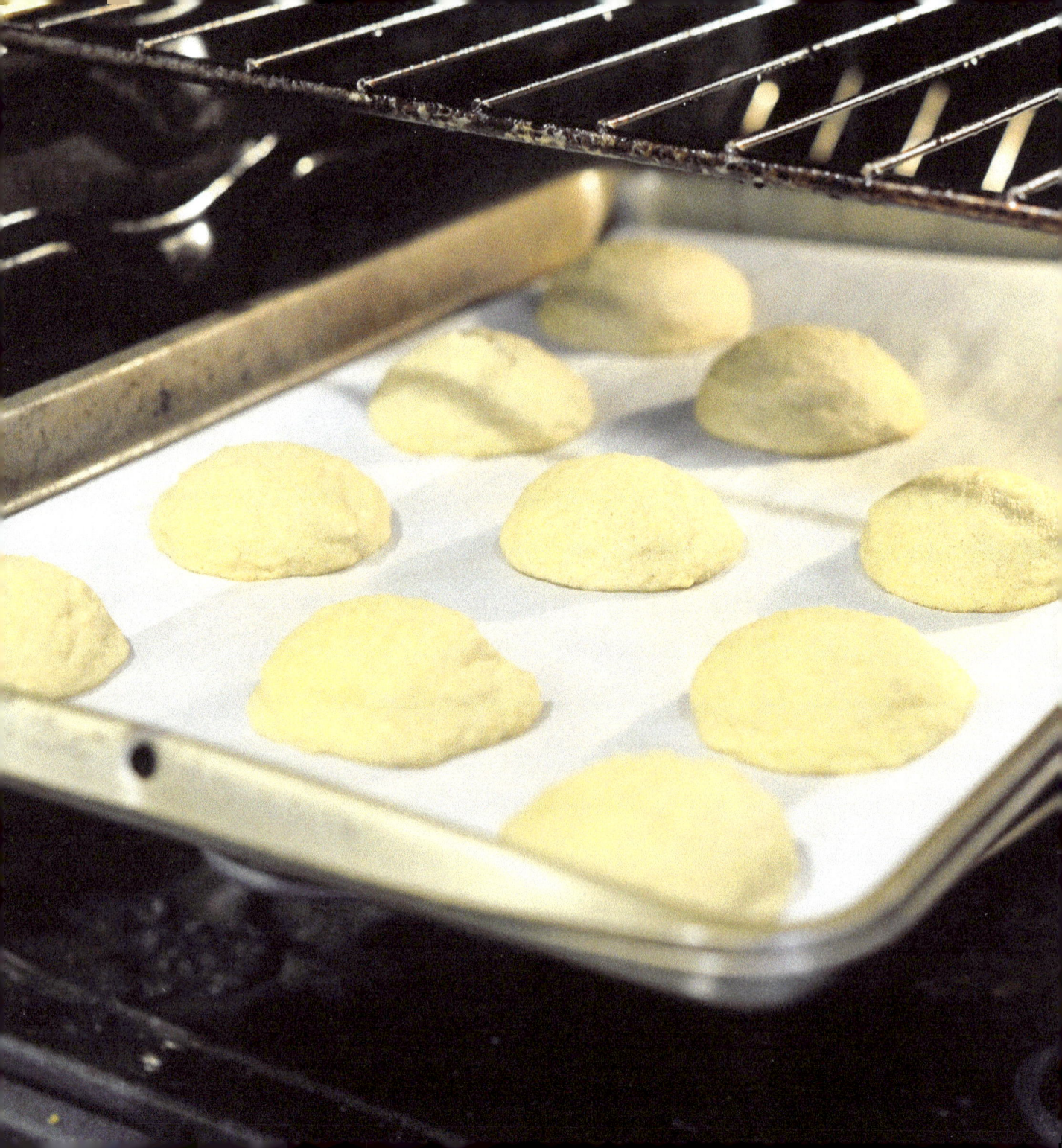

Dedicated to Ian, the nicest kid you'll ever meet, and to Aidan, the boy who couldn't have sugar.

Special thanks to Christine, JK, Jack, Irish, Kelly, Lisa, Margaux, and Orlando, our Personal Shopper Team from Whole Foods Market. You were all so amazing, and always willing to try the things we invented. Without you, this wouldn't be possible.

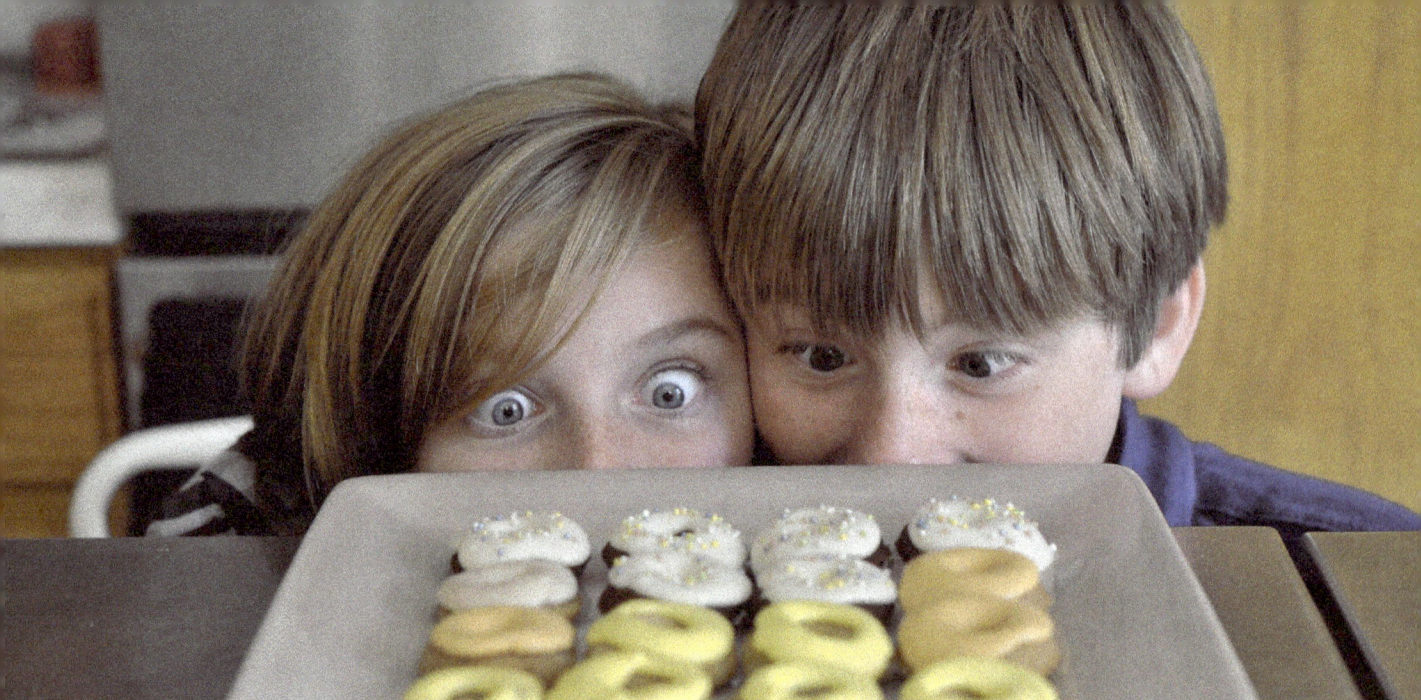

Designed, Edited, Produced, Directed, and Styled by the Free & Friendly Foods Team

US Library of Congress cataloging-in-publication data has been applied for.

ISBN 978-1-945374-00-5
© Copyright 2016

Disclaimer

The recipes in this book are not medical advice. Please consult with your doctor or allergist if necessary before trying any of these items. If you feel you are having a medical emergency seek help and dial 9-1-1.

Need Help?

We are always happy to help people with any questions they may have. If you're new to the food allergy community, or need help with a recipe, don't hesitate to reach out. Find us online at freeandfriendlyfoods.com. We also have a blog at foodandlego.com.

Contents

Introduction 11

Ingredients, Lingo, Tools 12

Tips 14

Substitutions 16

Helpful Chart 18

Cookies 20

Sauces, Chocolate, Candy 32

Cakes, Brownies, Muffins 38

Drinks 54

Pastries & Pies 58

Doughnuts 64

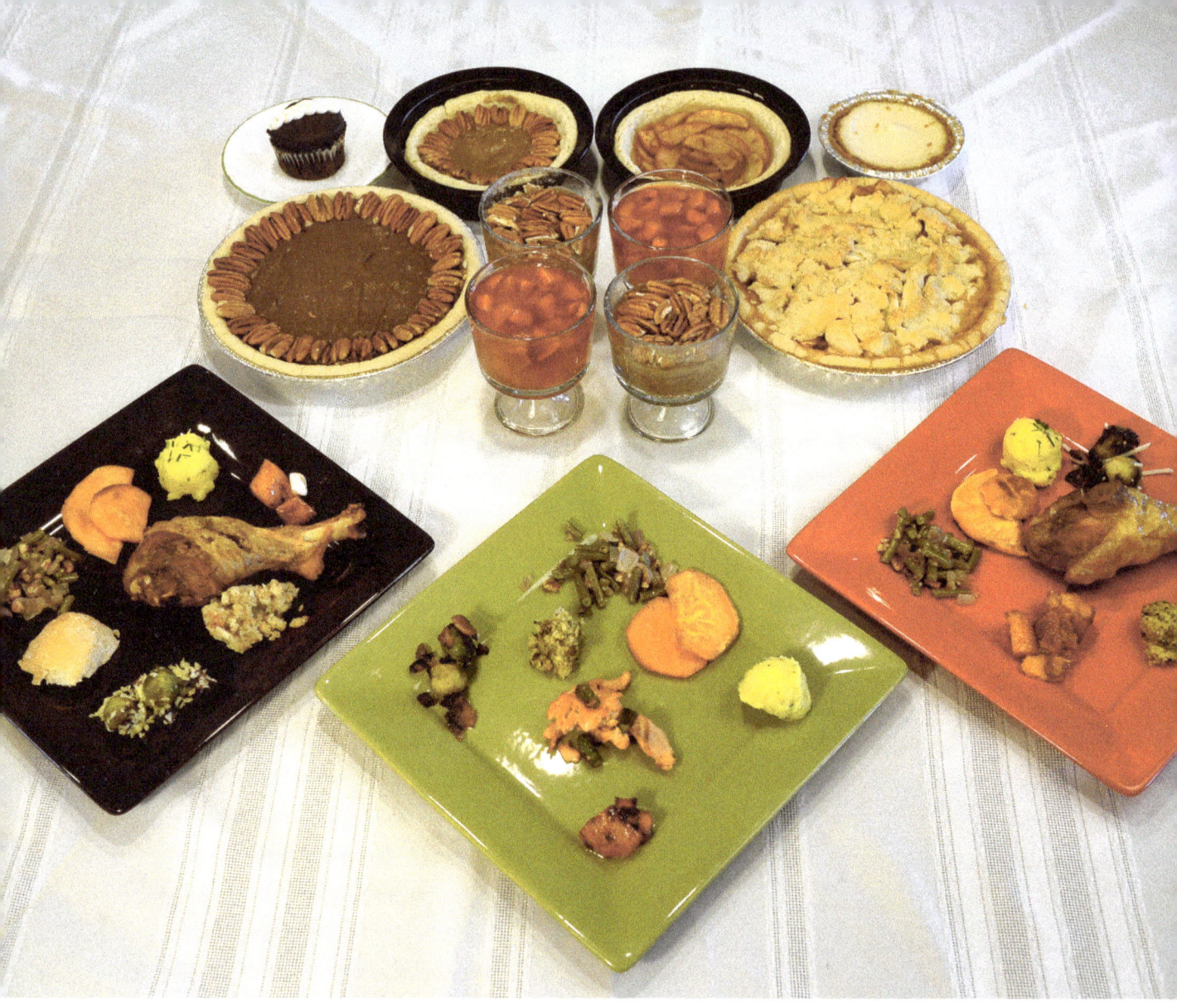

Conquering a very complicated Thanksgiving. Blend of Gluten Free, Dairy Free, Egg Free, Corn Free, Nut Free, Paleo Friendly, GAPs Friendly, and Low Sugar Foods. That's a mouth full...

Introduction

Welcome to the book! Our house has a unique story, and it's the reason this book exists. Of the 6 people in our household, 5 have allergies and/or restricted diets, and you'll love this, none of them are the same. Dad is allergic to coconut, and can have issues with macadamia nuts. Now, at a first glance, this doesn't seem like such a huge deal, in a shellfish sort of way. That's easy to avoid, right? Well, when you have to have dairy free, coconut is a common substitute. On to Kid One. He's on GAPs for a variety of reasons. He's also done juicing, and things like camel milk. Kid Two, he was born allergic to dairy. As he was growing up, I knew there was an issue, but couldn't put my finger on it. He had a great pediatrician who helped us diagnose his wheat allergy. Later, we learned that he had low vitamin D, and had developed a problem with eggs. At that point, we put him on a four-day food rotation, and went about reinventing the wheel for the fifth time. Enter Kid Three. He can't have processed and refined sugars, and can't have food coloring and pesticides. He eats organic, and I limit him to no more than 15g of added sugar per day. It can make some things like desserts tough, but he knows he gets small amounts because we care. Then there's Kid Four. She's totally OK. We all love to remember when she said to her brothers, "I wish I got to eat special food like you..." and they all shouted "NO!" at the same time. They told her how much they wished they could be like her. The grass is always greener I suppose. Lastly, there's me, The Allergy Chef. Turns out I had an undiagnosed set of food allergies and sensitivities. I ended up over 400 pounds, was coughing up blood daily, and was just too sick to function. Then, without notice, I started to have something like anaphylaxis responses, and couldn't eat much. Then water became an issue. Needless to say, we've had to learn so much about food, how it's made, what's really in it, and how to reinvent it. In these pages are little gems that we hope will bring smiles to your faces and warmth to your tummies. We hope our story helps you on your journey.

Common Ingredients

Flours & Baking
Sweet Sorghum Flour (Bob's Red Mill, BRM)
Potato Starch (BRM)
Tapioca Starch (BRM)
Organic Buckwheat Flour
Arrowroot Starch (BRM)**
Gluten Free Old Fashioned Rolled Oats (BRM)
Baking Powder (Hain Featherweight, corn free)
Baking Soda**

King Arthur Almond Flour, blanched*
Bob's Red Mill Blanched or Natural Almond Flour*

The Pure Pantry Dark Chocolate Cake Mix
King Arthur Gluten Free Cake Mix

Chocolates
Raw Organic Cacao Butter**
Enjoy Life Semi-sweet Chocolate Chips
Enjoy Life Dark Chocolate Chips
Raw Organic Cacao Powder**

Sweeteners
Raw Organic Sugar
Organic Sugar
Organic Powdered Sugar
Organic Light & Dark Brown Sugars
Organic Maple Sugar*
Organic Molasses
Raw Organic Honey (Y.S. Brand)*
Raw Organic Agave

Seasonings*
Sea Salt
Pink Himalayan Salt

Organic Ground Cinnamon
Organic Ground Nutmeg
Organic Ground Cloves
Organic Raw Ground Vanilla Bean

Extracts & Flavors
Organic Vanilla Extract
Organic Orange Flavoring
Organic Peppermint Flavor/Extract
Organic Lemon Flavor/Extract
Organic Almond Extract
Strawberry Flavor (Co-op Natural Brand)

India Tree Natural Colors

Milk & Butter
Organic Unsweetened Almond Milk*
Earth Balance Vegan Buttery Sticks
Organic Cream Cheese

Nuts & Seeds*
Organic Raw Cashews
Organic Raw Walnuts
Organic Raw Pecans
Organic Raw Brazil Nuts
Organic Raw Macadamia Nuts
Organic Chia Seeds (Black & White)

Dried Fruit
Organic Raw Medjool Dates*
Organic Golden Raisins*
Organic Black Raisins*
Organic Dried Cranberries, sweetened

*Indicates Paleo & GAPs Friendly
**Indicates Paleo Friendly
For strict Paleo & GAPs, extracts should be home-made

Lingo & Tools

Unless you're already a seasoned pro, there are several tools that you should become familiar with, and some common lingo we use throughout the book.

tsp & t are both short for teaspoon

TBSP & T are both short for Tablespoon. There are 3t in 1T.

c is short for cup.

GF = Gluten Free, DF = Dairy free, EF = Egg Free, NF = Nut Free, CF = Corn Free

Room Temp, usually referring to butter and eggs, means we allow it to sit out until it's no longer chilled. With butter, it should be easy to press with a finger (soft), but not melted.

Small and Medium Cookie Dough Scooper. We use the OXO brand, and they are simply awesome. The small scooper holds 2t and the medium holds 1.5T. There's also a large one, but we use an ice cream scooper for bigger scoops.

Good measuring cups and spoons. We like the OXO brand because it's accurate. Be sure to have dry measuring spoons, and something for liquids, such as Pyrex.

A good blender. We have a Vitamix. It's great for blending, easy to clean, and simply wonderful. When mixing lots of nuts and dates, something heavy duty will make your life much easier.

A good stand mixer. We have a Kitchen Aid. We simply couldn't live without ours. You can mix by hand, but this will make things go much faster.

Scissors. I use regularly to open packages, etc. We keep 2 sets for food items, 3 for baking, and 1 utility pair in the kitchen. Why so many? With all the allergies, we wash them after each use to prevent cross contamination.

Tips For The Recipes

Everything in the book can be made soy free.
We've had great experiences with Earth Balance Vegan Buttery Sticks, which contains soy. We prefer this brand because it's not made in a shared facility with dairy, which Kid Two is severely allergic to. To make the recipes soy free, use dairy-based butter if you can. If not, consider using Spectrum Shortening, but you may have a problem if you can't have coconut (cross reactions), and there have been some reactions reported by those allergic to corn. You can also experiment with olive oil, coconut oil, or Earth Balance Soy Free Sticks.

For those allergic to nuts, we use almond milk as a default.
All of the recipes can easily use soy, rice, or dairy milk, in addition to other milk alternatives. Avoid using water, unless you're corn, nut, and dairy allergic.

It's Simple so you CAN Substitute.
You may notice some of the recipes are simple, or don't use store-bought flour blends. That's done to make them easy to change. We know that no two people with allergies are the same, so we encourage you to change things when necessary.

The other reason this was done was to aid in a 4-day food rotation for Kid Two. Those of you with particular allergy conditions know all about 4 day rotations. In our case, I needed Kid Two to be able to eat actual rice on day 1, and cookies on day 4. This meant no rice flour at all.

Prep, Freeze, and Freeze!
Many of the recipes can be frozen and used again later. Sometimes, it's the batter that you freeze, other times, the whole dish. If you have more than one child, or live a busy life, this will become an awesome part of your kitchen routine. Fun tip for freezing: baked items that contain rice based flours freeze well, but don't thaw as well all the time. Keep that in mind if you're freezing muffins or cookies that contain rice.

Parchment Paper and Muffin Cup Liners are your new best friends.

When we first got into gluten and dairy free baking, and later egg free, I couldn't figure out why our recipes would consistently stick to the pans. It especially happened if I tried to make something corn free. At times, it was only a little stick. Other times, you had to put some major elbow grease into it when releasing the item. I was using non-stick pans. Was this false advertising?! No, it wasn't. I learned the hard way that manufactures produce their products with the majority of their users in mind, not the small percentage that can't (or won't) use mainstream ingredients. After many messes, I decided to try using parchment paper, and presto! Everything was peachy, golden, and any other word that represents happiness. This discovery also led me to use muffin liners for EVERYTHING. No really. Anything and everything I could think of, and it's been nothing but success, and easy clean ups.

We don't grease anything

In traditional baking, you grease pans. I found that when doing this with GF DF baking, it didn't help anything. You can experiment with non-stick sprays. We use it from time to time when someone is around to spray pans outside for me since they contain corn.

All About Substitutions - Eggs & Dairy

Eggs are a common ingredient in baking, and it's important to know why. Eggs are a binder, can be used as a leavening agent, and can also add moisture to your recipe. Not only are they nutritious, they help hold ingredients together. If you can't have eggs, here are several options that all "equal" one egg. I'll come back to those quotes in a moment.

1 TBSP Ground Flax + 3 TBSP Water
1 TBSP Chia Seeds + 1/3 cup Water
1 TBSP Soy Protein + 3 TBSP Water
1 TBSP Agar Agar + 1 TBSP Water
2 TBSP Arrowroot Flour
2 TBSP Potato Starch
1/2 Ripe, Smashed Banana
1/4 cup Unsweetened Applesauce
3 TBSP Peanut Butter
Commercial egg replacer such as Ener-G or Daiya brands

These should "equal" and egg, but in all honesty, they never really do. As you get into EF baking, especially if you are also DF and GF, things just don't work the way conventional recipes do. Our kids have gotten use to cookies that crumble, and simply accept this as a fact of life.

All About Substitutions - Dairy

Dairy is a common ingredient in baking and cooking. Cow's milk is creamy, and doesn't have much flavor. This makes it very useful for sweet and savory cooking and baking. What makes it better than water is the texture, and general makeup.

Dairy substitutions are simple. You can use rice, soy, almond, hemp, hazelnut, and coconut milk alternatives. Rice milk is thin. Beware. Soy is close to the thickness of milk, but we don't like it given the soy issues in this country. Almond milk works well, and we prefer to use organic unsweetened almond milk. Hemp is simply odd in taste. Hazelnut milk has a strong flavor, so it may not work well in all recipes. Coconut milk is nice and thick. It can work well, but does have a distinct flavor unlike some of the other choices. More than anything, experiment and see which one you like best!

All About Substitutions - Wheat

A note about how we use flour. As previously mentioned, Kid Two requires a special food rotation, so when putting together new recipes for him, I purposefully used single flours, rather than a blend. Most GF flours contain rice, which we needed to avoid, so he could eat rice with other meals. If you don't need a rotation, you should try using your normal flour in place of ours, and you will most likely have even better results. Part of the reason the store-bought blends work is because of the texture combinations, as well as the xantham gum etc. that's added. For us, with my severe corn allergy, xantham gum usually isn't allowed in the house.

To All of "My People" With a Corn Allergy

If corn is your only allergy, then you'll need to source safe eggs and dairy. If you have a severe corn allergy, you may find that eating the products of animals fed corn can cause problems for you, even though "it's not supposed to." You may reach a point where you need to do lots of research to find safe farms in your area. You may also be able to find a farmer willing to mail you frozen goods. If you live in the PA area, the Amish are an amazing resource. There are also great farms in Oregon.

If you have mixed allergies with corn, you may be better off making your own almond milk if you don't have a nut allergy. Be sure to use a corn free nut milk bag. If you can't have eggs or corn, the potato starch and chia seed method still works, however, you'll need to find safe potato starch and chia. Bob's Red Mill is great for GF people, and hit-or-miss for CF people.

One final CF note... there are many recipes that may look corn free compatible that I haven't listed as such. I did this based on the odds of you finding safe ingredients. It doesn't mean it can't be done. It's more of a question of how bad do you want this treat?

The Chart... As Requested by The Papa

If you know me well, you know I hate the index in the back of a cookbook. I don't know why, I just do. So, when The Papa insisted there be one, I said Nope. Then he reexplained what he really meant, and I loved the idea. So, here's The Papa's chart to make finding what you need a lot easier.

Recipe	Page	Freeze Well	GF	DF	EF	NF	CF	Soy Free	Paleo	GAPs
Oatmeal Cookies	20	✳ ✳	✓	✓	✓	✳	✗	✳	✗	✗
Honey Orange Ginger Cookies	23	✳ ✳	✓	✓	✓	✓	✳	✳	✗	✗
Peanut Butter Chocolate Chip Cookies	24	✳ ✳	✓	✓	✓	✗	✗	✳	✗	✗
Citrus Cloud Cookies	27	✳ ✳	✓	✓	✓	✳	✗	✳	✗	✗
Paleo Thumbprint Cookie	28	✗	✓	✓	✓	✗	✓	✓	✓	✓
Apple Pie Cookie	31	✗	✓	✓	✗	✓	✓	✓	✓	✓
Caramel Sauce	32	✗	✓	✓	✓	✳	✗	✳	✗	✗
Filled Chocolates	35	✓	✓	✓	✓	✓	✗	✓	✗	✗
White Chocolate	36	✓	✓	✓	✓	✗	✓	✓	✓	✓
Caramel Nut Brownies	39	✓	✓	✓	✓	✳	✗	✳	✗	✗
Blueberry Lemon Loaf	40	✗	✓	✓	✓	✗	✓	✓	✓	✓
Lemon Lime Mini Muffins	43	✗	✓	✓	✓	✗	✓	✓	✓	✓
Pumpkin Puffs	44	✗	✓	✓	✓	✳	✗	✳	✗	✗
Spicy Icing	46	✗	✓	✓	✓	✓	✗	✳	✗	✗
Ginger Icing	47	✗	✓	✓	✓	✓	✗	✳	✗	✗

GF = Gluten Free   DF = Dairy Free   EF = Egg Free   NF = Nut Free   CF = Corn Free

Recipe	Page	Freeze Well	GF	DF	EF	NF	CF	Soy Free	Paleo	GAPs
Graham Cracker Crunch Icing	48	✗	✓	✓	✓	✓	✗	✗	✗	✗
Creme Cookie Crunch Cupcakes	49	✗	✓	✓	✓	✓	✗	✗	✗	✗
Cream Filled Strawberry Cupcake	50	✗	✓	✓	✓	✓	✗	✳	✗	✗
Peppermint Icing	51	✗	✓	✓	✓	✓	✗	✳	✗	✗
Banana Cream Cheese Icing	52	✗	✓	✓	✓	✓	✗	✳	✗	✗
Peanut Butter Icing	53	✗	✓	✓	✓	✗	✳	✳	✗	✗
Cashew Chocolate Smoothie	54	✗	✓	✓	✓	✗	✳	✓	✓	✓
Spinach Blueberry Smoothie	55	✗	✓	✓	✓	✗	✗	✓	✓	✓
Strawberry Cashew Smoothie	56	✗	✓	✓	✓	✗	✗	✓	✓	✓
Tropical Ice Cream	57	✓	✓	✓	✓	✓	✗	✓	✓	✓
Paleo Fruit Pastry	58	✗	✓	✓	✓	✗	✓	✓	✓	✓
Jam Filled Pastry	59	✗	✓	✓	✓	✓	✗	✳	✗	✗
Stuffed Apple Cups	60	✗	✓	✓	✓	✳	✳	✓	✓	✓
Fudgey Banana Date Pie	63	✗	✓	✓	✓	✳	✗	✓	✓	✗
Cinnamon Doughnuts	67	✳✳	✓	✓	✓	✳	✗	✳	✗	✗
Chocolate Doughnuts	68	✳✳	✓	✓	✓	✳	✗	✳	✗	✗
Cake Doughnuts	71	✳✳	✓	✓	✓	✳	✗	✳	✗	✗
Maple Doughnuts	72	✳✳	✓	✓	✓	✳	✗	✳	✗	✗

✓ Good to Go   ✗ No Go   ✳ ✳ Batter/Raw Materials Only   ✳ Modifications Needed

Chewy Oatmeal Cookies

Gluten, Dairy, Egg Free

Soy Free Compatible, Optionally nut free, but texture and taste will change

These have received rave reviews from "normal" eaters as well as the allergy community. Their best feature is shelf life; after 5 days, they're still great. The kids keep eating them, so I don't know about day 6.

Soy Free Compatible: Use safe butter.

Ingredients:

2 (16T) Sticks Dairy Free Butter, room temp.

1/4 cup Organic Dark Brown Sugar

1/2 cup Organic White Sugar

2/3 cup Organic Walnuts (crushed/small pieces)

1/3 cup Organic Pecans (crushed/small pieces)

5 TBSP Organic Sweetened Cranberries

1 TBSP Organic Vanilla Extract

4 TBSP Organic Raisins

4 tsp Baking Powder

1/2 tsp Sea Salt

3 TBSP Potato Starch

2 TBSP Organic Black Chia Seeds

2/3 cup Organic Almond Milk (or milk of choice)

1 1/2 cup Certified GF Rolled Oats

1 cup White Sorghum Flour

Directions:

Combine the milk, chia seeds, and potato starch, and set aside.

Next, cream the butter and sugars together in a mixing bowl on medium speed. Add in the dried fruit and nuts, and mix again. Next, add the baking powder, and milk/seed/starch mix. Allow it to fizz and rise for 2 minutes. Add in all of the other ingredients and mix until it's well incorporated.

Using a large dough scooper or ice cream scooper, scoop large mounds on to a cookie sheet lined with parchment paper.

Bake at 325 for 15 minutes. After baking, move the parchment paper and cookies onto a surface to cool.

Experiment with how much to press down your dough mounds. This will effect how soft and doughy the center of the cookie is.

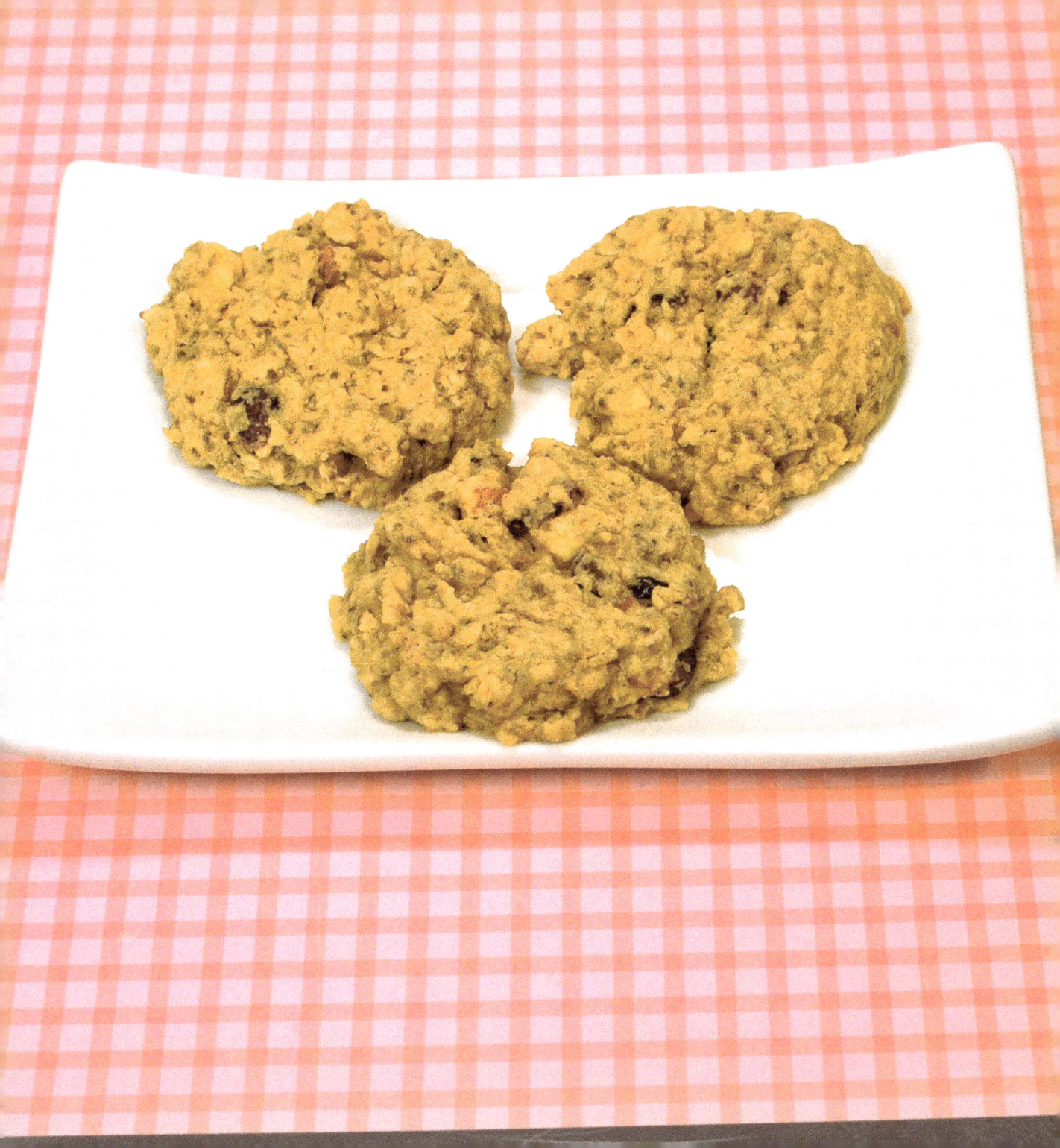

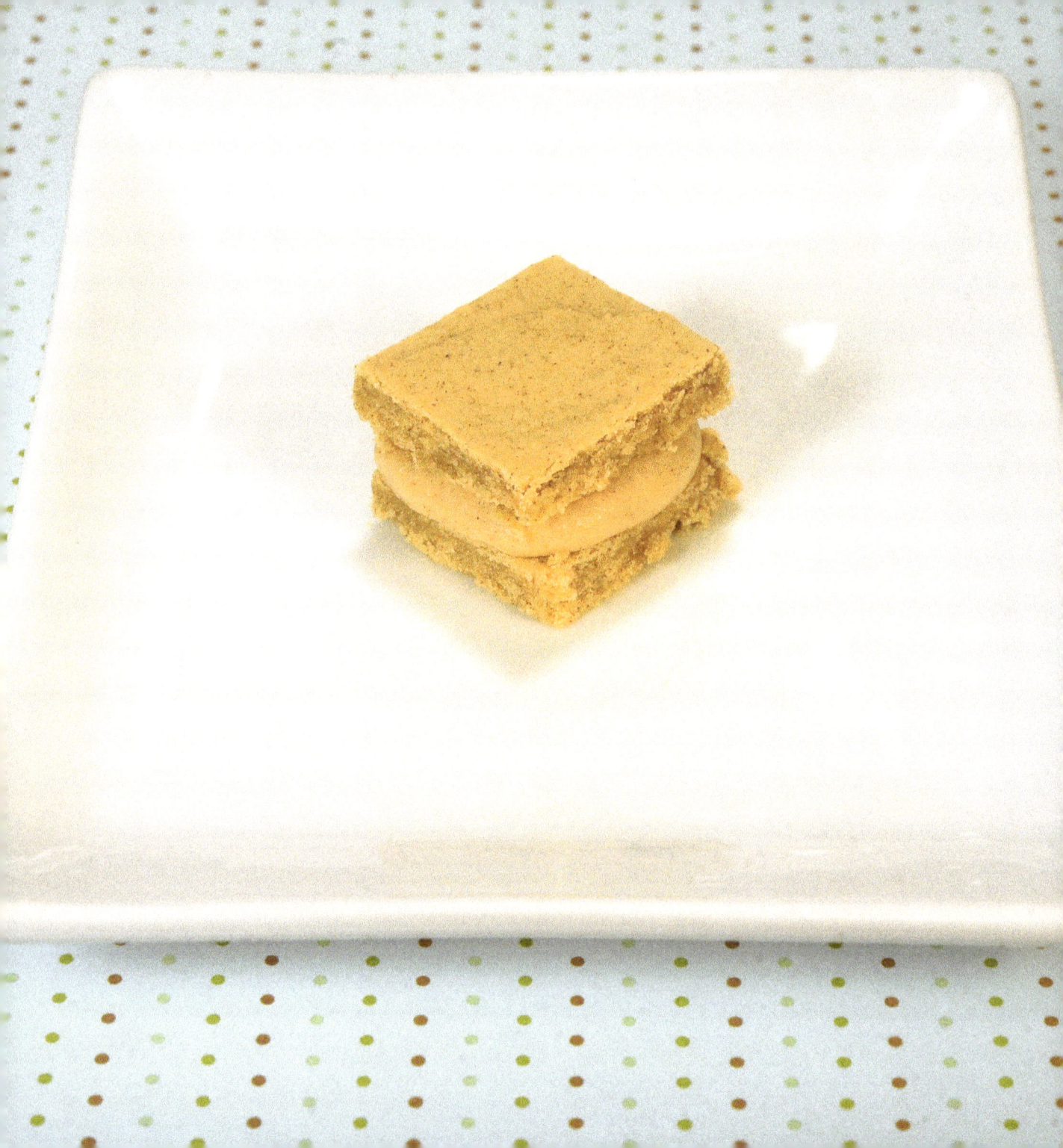

Orange Honey Ginger Cookies

Gluten, Dairy, Egg, Nut Free
Corn & Soy Free Compatible

Corn Free Compatible: Use safe ingredients. Hain Baking Powder is CF. You may need to make your own vanilla extract, or use ground vanilla bean instead. For orange flavoring, use the zest of a safe orange.
Soy Free Compatible: Use safe butter.

Ingredients:

2 Sticks (16T) Dairy Free Butter, room temp.

1 cup Organic Honey

1/2 tsp Sea Salt

1/8 tsp Organic Ground Ginger

      (use 1/4 tsp for more "bite")

1 1/2 tsp Organic Ground Cinnamon

1/4 tsp Organic Ground Nutmeg

4 tsp Baking Powder

1 TBSP Organic Vanilla Extract

1 tsp Organic Orange Flavoring/Extract

6 TBSP Potato Starch

2 1/3 cup White Sorghum Flour

Directions:

Cream the butter and sugar together in a mixing bowl on medium speed. Next, add in everything but the flour and mix well until it's all incorporated. Lastly, add in the flour and mix again until a dough forms.

Bake at 350 for 16 minutes for standard cookies, and 13 minutes as a large flat cookie sheet (cookie-bar).

Fun Idea! Makes a cookie sandwich! Bake the dough flat on a cookie sheet (cookie bar) with parchment paper. Cut cookie squares and add icing in between two cookie squares. The shelf life of the sandwich is 5 days (or more) in an air-tight container. After 10 days, we found that it was still edible, but only the icing and lower level of the cookie. The top had become too hard/stale.

Peanut Butter Chocolate Chip Cookies

Gluten, Dairy, Egg Free
Soy Free Compatible

Ingredients:

2 Sticks (16T) Dairy Free Butter, room temp.

1 cup Organic Peanut Butter

1 cup Organic Cane Sugar, white

1/2 cup Organic Light Brown Sugar

1 tsp Sea Salt

3 tsp Baking Powder

3 tsp Organic Vanilla Extract

6 TBSP Potato Starch

3 cups Sweet White Sorghum Flour

3/4 cup Organic Unsweetened Almond Milk

1 cup Enjoy Life Chocolate Chips

Directions:

Cream the butter, peanut butter, and sugars together on high speed. Scrape the edges and cream again to ensure it's well mixed. Add in all of the ingredients, except for the flour and mix again. Last, add in the flour and pulse the mixer to start the blending, then turn up to medium-high speed until a dough forms.

Bake at 350 for 12 minutes. Cooks well from a fresh and chilled dough.

Soy Free Compatible: Use safe butter.

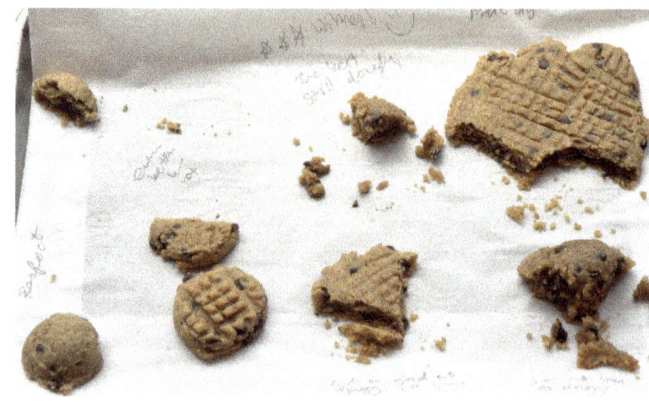

We made a "cookie map" to determine how much to flatten the dough before baking. Here are the results:

- Small dough scoop, unflattened, is perfect
- Small dough scoop, flattened is even better
- Medium dough scoop, flattened, not as good as the doughy ones, but still good
- Extra large scoop, flattened, came out dry
- Winner: Medium scoop, unflattened. It's doughy in the middle and tastes great!

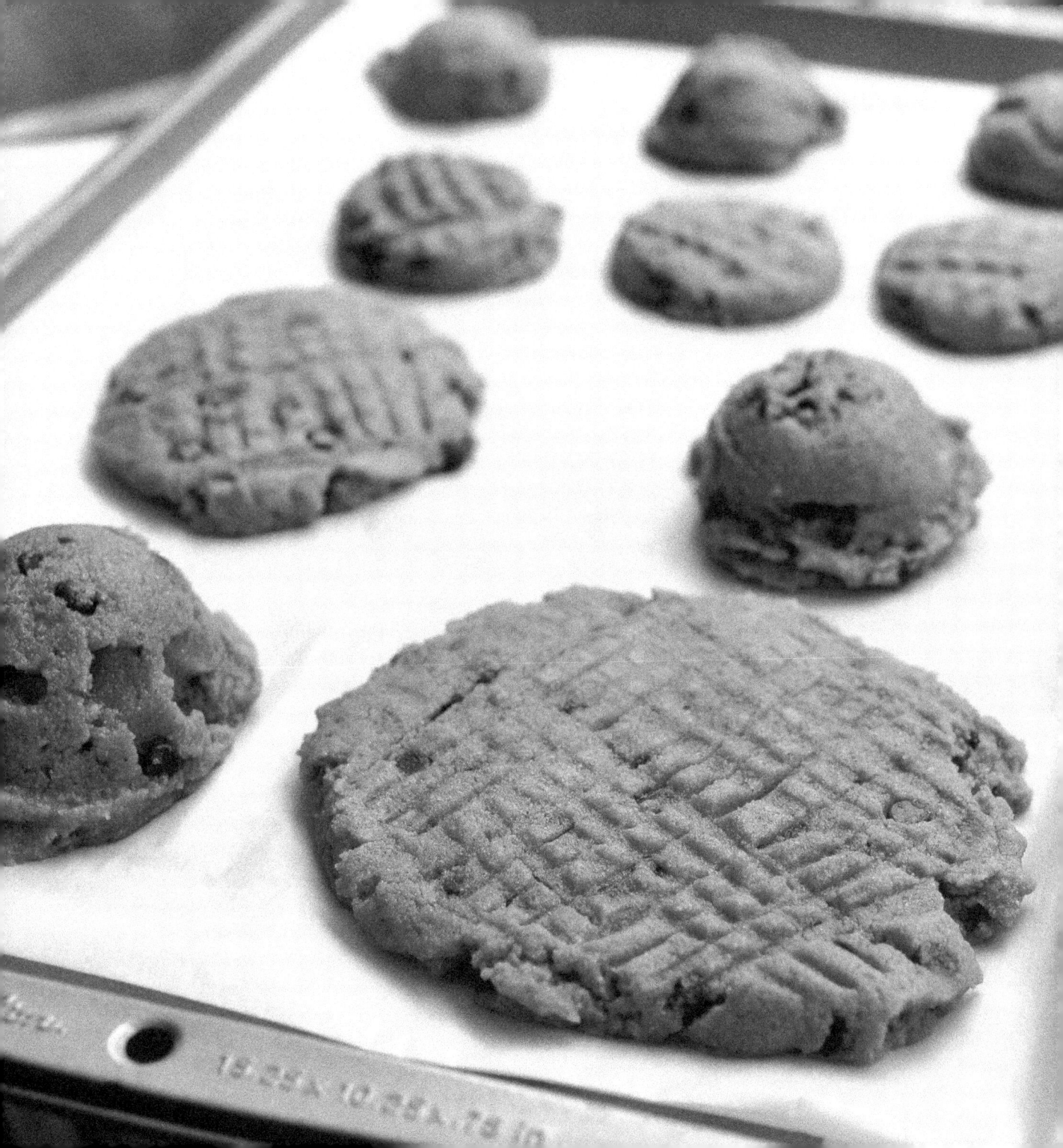

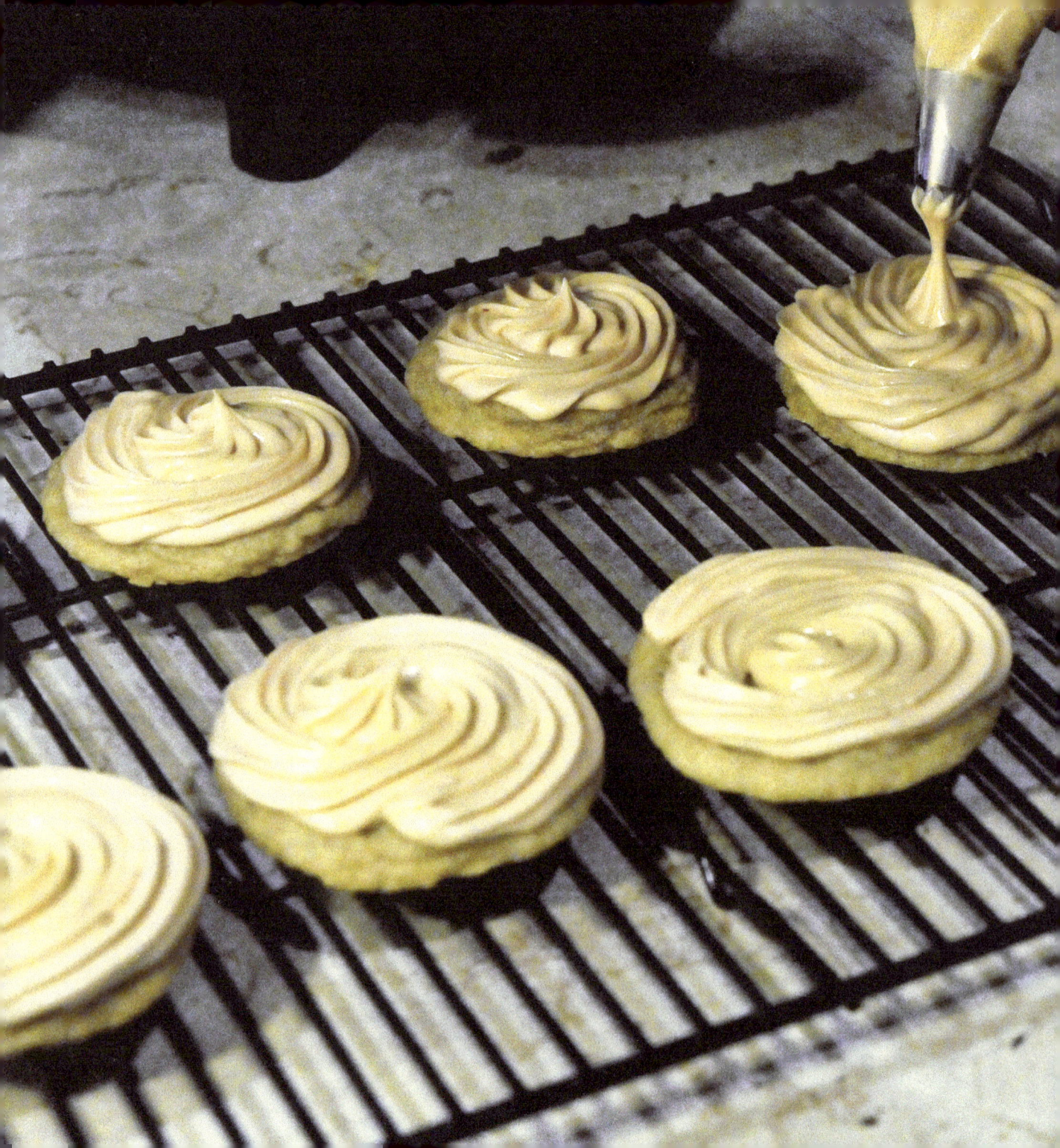

Citrus Cloud Cookies

Gluten, Dairy, Egg Free
Soy & Nut Free Compatible

The goal when creating this cookie was to end up with a scrumptious edible cloud. After several different variations (and lots of taste testing), we reached success!

Ingredients:

2 1/2 Sticks (20T) Dairy Free Butter, room temp.

1 cup Organic Cane Sugar

3/4 tsp Organic Lemon Extract/Flavoring

2 tsp Organic Vanilla Extract

5 tsp Baking Powder

1/4 tsp Sea Salt

5 TBSP Potato Starch

1/3 cup organic unsweetened almond milk

2 1/2 cups White Sorghum Flour

Silky Icing

1 Stick Dairy Free Butter (8T), room temp.

4 cups Organic Powdered Sugar (1 standard bag)

2 tsp Organic Vanilla Extract

1/8 tsp Sea Salt

1/2 tsp Organic Orange Extract/Flavoring

3 TBSP + 2 tsp Water

Red & Yellow India Tree Natural Colors
(add a bit more water, 1t at a time if you omit color)

Directions:

Combine the milk and potato starch and set aside. Cream the butter and sugar together on medium-high speed. Scrape down the edges, and add in the rest of the items (including the milk and potato starch), except for the flour. Wait 2 minutes to give the baking powder time to work its magic. Add in your flour and mix until a dough forms. Don't over-mix. You could upset the delicate balance of the cloud.

Bake at 350 for 10 minutes. Cool on the hot cookie sheet for 2 minutes, then remove to a flat surface. This dough does not cook well from cold, so be sure it's at room temperature. Baking on parchment paper makes it easier to release the cookies.

Once the cookies have cooled, dot or swirl with the silky icing. Some felt the swirl was a bit too sweet, others didn't. You have to know your audience for this one. The cookies stay moist and delicious for several days, even uncovered.

Soy Free Compatible: Use safe butter.
Nut Free Compatible: Use safe milk.

Paleo Thumbprint Cookie

Gluten, Dairy, Egg, Soy, Corn Free
Paleo & GAPs Friendly

These cookies were inspired by Sugar Plum Vegan. They introduced a Paleo thumbprint which got the ideas flowing. Eating these warm is a real treat, and eating them cool is still a great treat.

Ingredients:

1 cup Blanched Almond Flour

1/8 tsp Pink Himalayan Salt

4 tsp Organic Coconut Oil

1/4 cup Organic Maple Butter

Fruit Filling

1 Large Organic Peach (or fruit of choice)

2 TBSP Organic Black Chia Seeds

Notes:

Personally, I found these to be a bit on the sweet side, too much for me. Everyone else thought they were perfect. I also found that without the filling, this is still an awesome cookie.

Directions:

Blend the Peach until it's very liquidy, then stir in the chia seeds. Set aside and allow the seeds to expand.

Mix the dough ingredients together. It may be easier to use your hand. Roll a spoon of dough in your hands into a ball, and flatten on a cookie sheet that has parchment paper. Using a spoon, flatten the center of the dough more to create a cavity for the fruit mix. Repeat until the dough is all gone. Spoon in the peach mix. You can use as little or as much as you'd like, but try not to overflow the cookie.

Bake at 350 for 10 minutes. Cool on the hot cookie sheet for 3 minutes. Remove the parchment and cookies from the cookie sheet and cool on a flat surface.

This makes 4 good sized cookies, and there's a little dough for sampling.

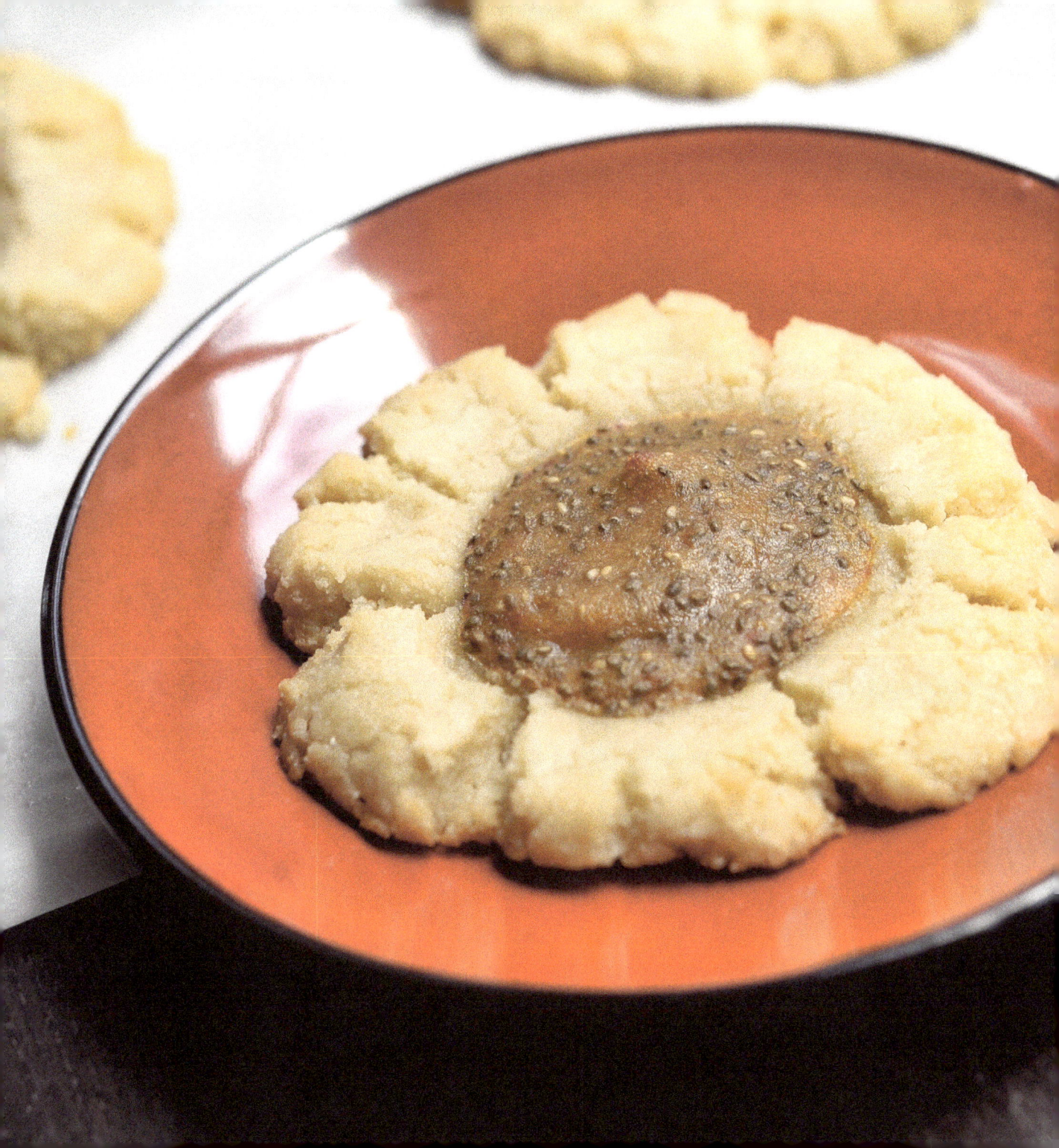

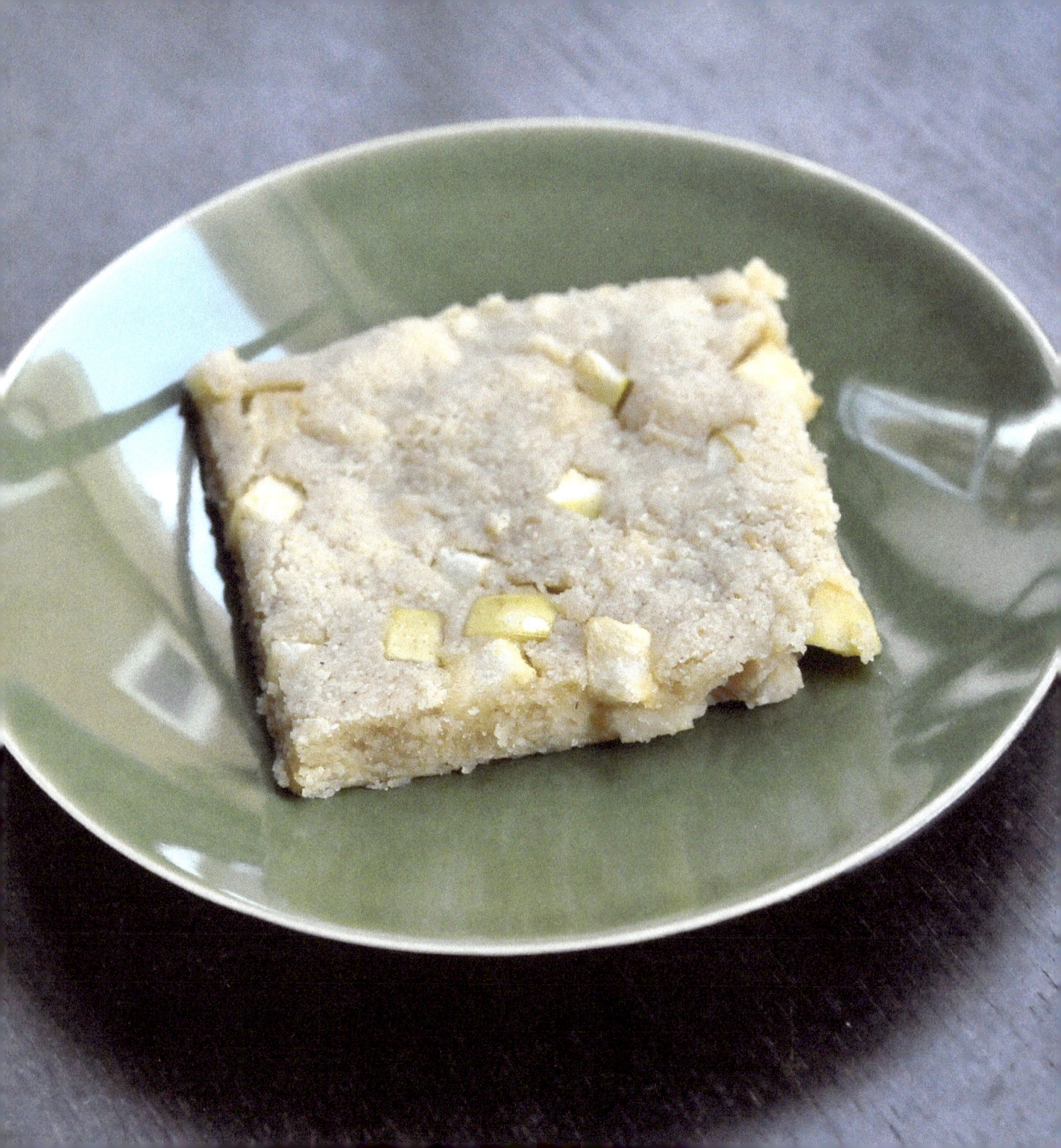

Apple Pie Cookie

Gluten, Dairy, Egg, Soy, Corn Free
Paleo & GAPs Friendly

After having no treats for years, this was like eating the most delicious slice of apple pie of all time. I don't recommend this if you aren't eating Paleo and GAPs regularly as it may seem foreign to you.

Ingredients:

2 cups Blanched Almond Flour

1/4 tsp Organic Ground Nutmeg

3/4 tsp Organic Ground Cinnamon

1/4 tsp Pink Himalayan Salt

6 tsp Organic Coconut Oil

2.5 Medium Cookie Dough Scoop Organic Maple Butter, approx. 3.5T

3/4 of an Organic Gravenstein Apple, small cubed pieces

If you have a corn allergy, be sure to source safe, local apples that are free of pesticides, and know how they're grown. I've found one local grower that has proven to be safe.

Directions:

Mix everything but the apple together. It may be easier to use your hand. If you store your coconut oil in the fridge, bring it to room temperature first if you use a mixer. If you use your hand, the heat will soften it quickly. Once everything is together, add in the apples and mix a bit more. Place the dough on parchment paper and press into a large "bar".

Bake at 350 for 10 minutes. Cool on the cookie sheet for 3 minutes. Remove the cookies and paper from the tray and cool on a flat surface.

Eat cool, warm, or uncooked. It's all delicious.

Caramel Sauce

Gluten, Dairy, Egg Free
Soy & Nut Free Compatible

Soy Free Compatible: Use safe butter.
Nut Free Compatible: Use safe milk.

I never knew that traditional caramel had dairy in it until I wanted to give some to the kids. At that point, I knew I had to figure it out. Caramel sauce almost didn't make it. Our early attempts were goopy and all wrong. After lots of research and development, I proudly present you with caramel sauce that's easy and enjoyable.

Ingredients:

1/2 cup Organic Light Brown Sugar

1/2 cup Organic Sugar

1/4 cup water

1 Stick Dairy Free Butter (8T)

1/3 cup Organic Unsweetened Almond Milk

4 Tbsp Potato Starch
(5 for thicker sauce for dipping or filling chocolates)

Directions:

Bring the water and sugar to a boil to allow the sugar to dissolve. As the mix starts to bubble and rise, turn the heat to low (3/10). Add in the other ingredients and whisk away like there's no tomorrow. When the butter melts, turn the heat off and continue to mix. As it cools, it will thicken up a bit more. For a thicker sauce, add more starch.

To make mini caramel apples (pictured), use a melon baller to create apple bites from an organic green apple. Insert a stick, dip and twirl through the sauce, and top with whatever you'd like.
We used Let's Do Organic brand sprinkles, and Kinnikinnick crushed creme cookies, as well as India Tree brand decorating sugar.

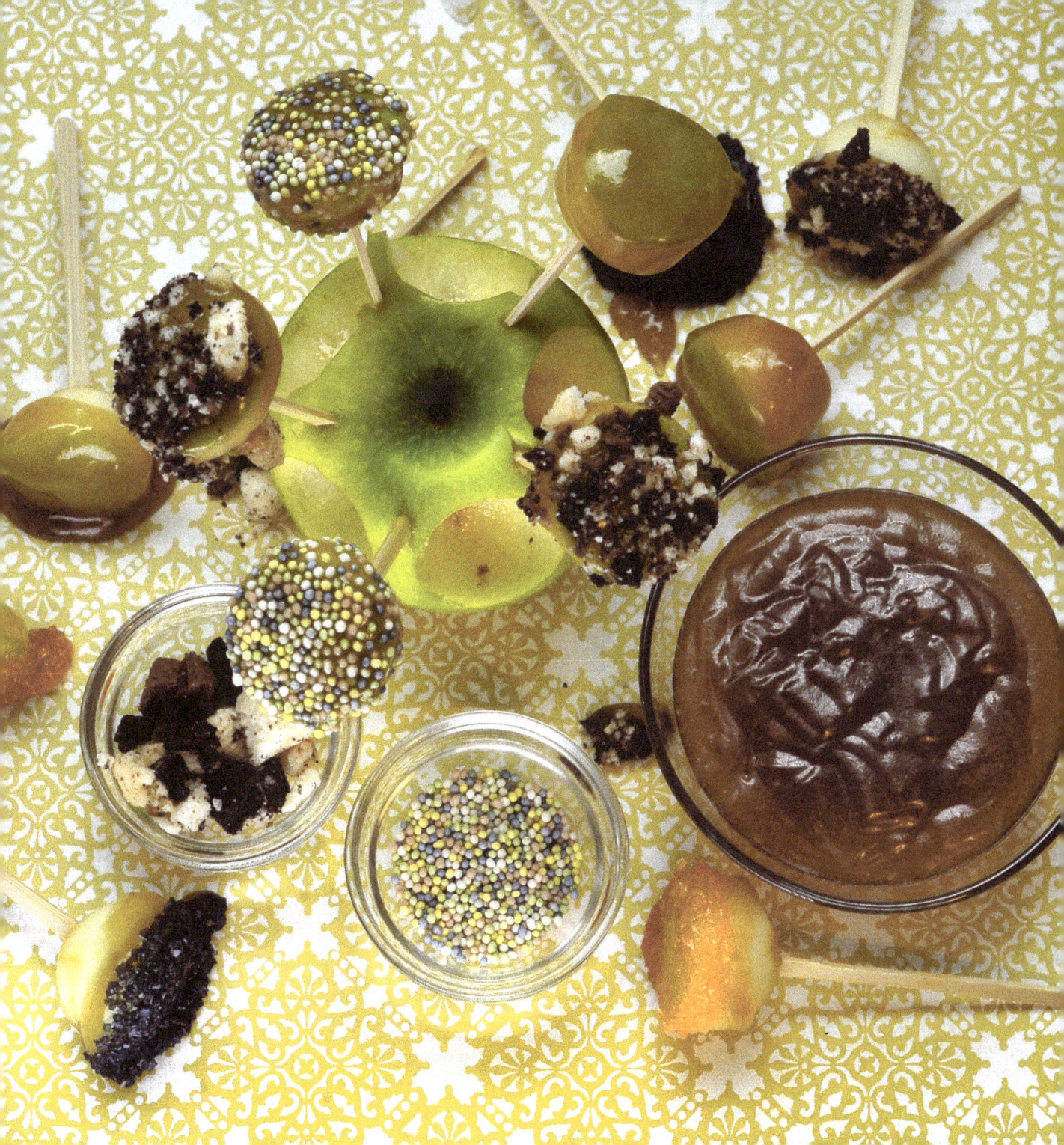

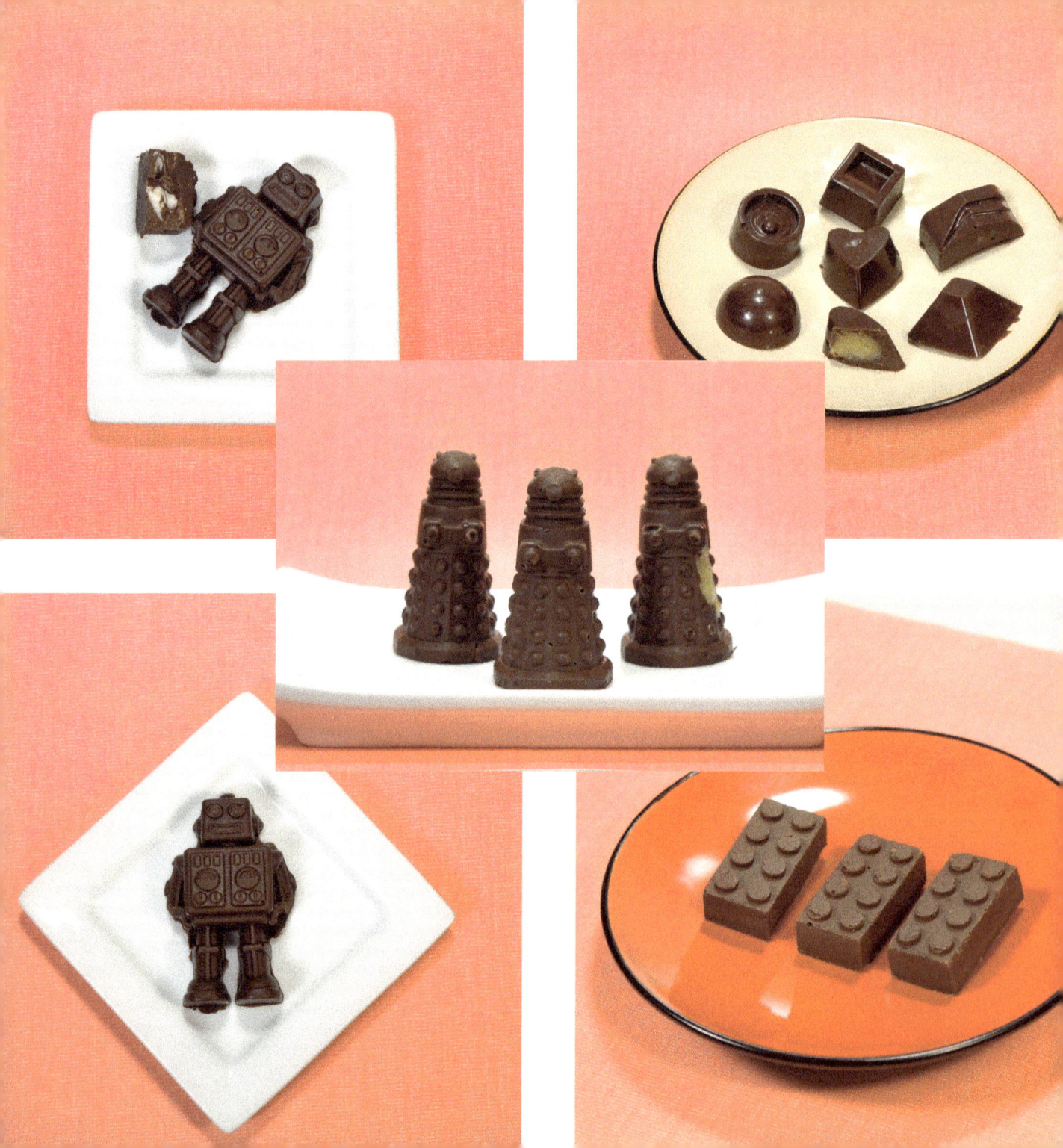

Caramel & Candy Filled Chocolates

Gluten, Dairy, Egg, Nut, Soy Free

Chocolate lovers, it is time to celebrate! After having problems with "chocolate bloom" I reached out to Enjoy Life, and they were SO helpful. They passed on so many tips that I want to share with you about melting and reforming their chocolate. Their chocolate does well when tempered, and starts to melt at 86 degrees, and shouldn't go over 115 degrees (f). For better results, and to help prevent bloom, add 1 - 2 tsp vegetable oil or shortening per bag that you melt. Counter-top setting will work to a degree, but these will shape better in the fridge or freezer. However, quick extreme changes in temperatures can cause poor results. They also wanted you to know that you can call and ask for help anytime. How cool!

Important Tools:

Double Boiler

Disposable Icing Bags or Chocolate Pouring Tool

Silicone Molds (Freshware are AMAZING)

Ingredients:

1 Bag Enjoy Life Chocolate Chips

Caramel Sauce or Candy Canes

You can use any hard candy, or get creative with your sauce. A fudge sauce or orange sauce would work well. Have FUN with these.

For caramel sauce, we used the recipe on the previous page, but added an extra TBSP of milk and tsp of potato starch to make it a bit thicker. We were also using it from the fridge, so it had already set. If you're making any sauce fresh, be mindful of how runny it will be when bitten into.

Directions:

In a double boiler, melt the chocolate chips. Stir occasionally, and a lot when they're almost smooth. I started with 3/4t oil and did OK.

Place an icing bag inside a tall glass cup to hold it in place to protect your hands from burning. Pour in the melted chocolate. Cut the tip and begin to fill your molds. This is a two person job. As you fill, have someone else use a toothpick to "raise" the chocolate around the edges of your mold. Fill the molds half way. I wear an oven mitt if I'm not using the chocolate pouring tool.

Add your filling. Use an icing bag for sauces. For crushed candy, simply sprinkle in. Cover with more chocolate.

Chill in the fridge (or freezer for faster treats). The Freshware molds release the chocolates by far the best. Other novelty molds are good, but small bits can break off easily.

White Chocolate

Gluten, Dairy, Egg, Soy, Corn Free
Paleo & GAPs Friendly

Currently, there's only one DF white chocolate that we've found on the market, but it's quite expensive. So, we've taken to making our own. It's cost effective, and freezes really well.

Important Tools:

Double Boiler (for small batches, and remelting)

Disposable Icing Bags or Chocolate Pouring Tool

Silicone Molds or Muffin Liners

Ingredients:

32 ounces Raw Organic Cacao Butter

1 cup Organic Maple Syrup
(If you're not Paleo or GAPs, you can add more)

1 1/2 cup Raw Organic Cashews

3/4 tsp Raw Organic Ground Vanilla

1/8 tsp Pink Salt, optional

Optional colors and flavor extracts if you're not Paleo/GAPs.

This is a basic mix that you can add color and flavor to. For St. Patrick's Day, we added green color (India Tree) and a little peppermint extract for something festive.

Directions:

This is what I consider to be a large fresh batch, so use a pot. If you're melting down a previously made batch, or making a very small batch, use a double boiler.

Start by melting the cacao butter on low heat (3/10). Once it's completely melted, transfer to your blender. Add in the other ingredients and mix on high speed until it's all smooth. Try to avoid having little bits of cashew in the mix.

Yield: 5 2/3 cups of white chocolate base.

This is where the fun starts. We divide our mix in to 6 or 8 parts, then add flavor and color to the parts. We've tried plain, creme cookie crunch, peppermint, strawberry, banana, coffee, lemon, and orange. Peppermint, Orange, Strawberry, and creme cookie have been the crowd favorites.

Place your chocolate in muffin liners or molds and freeze to allow it to set. Store in the freezer for whenever you'd like to use them, or eat right away.

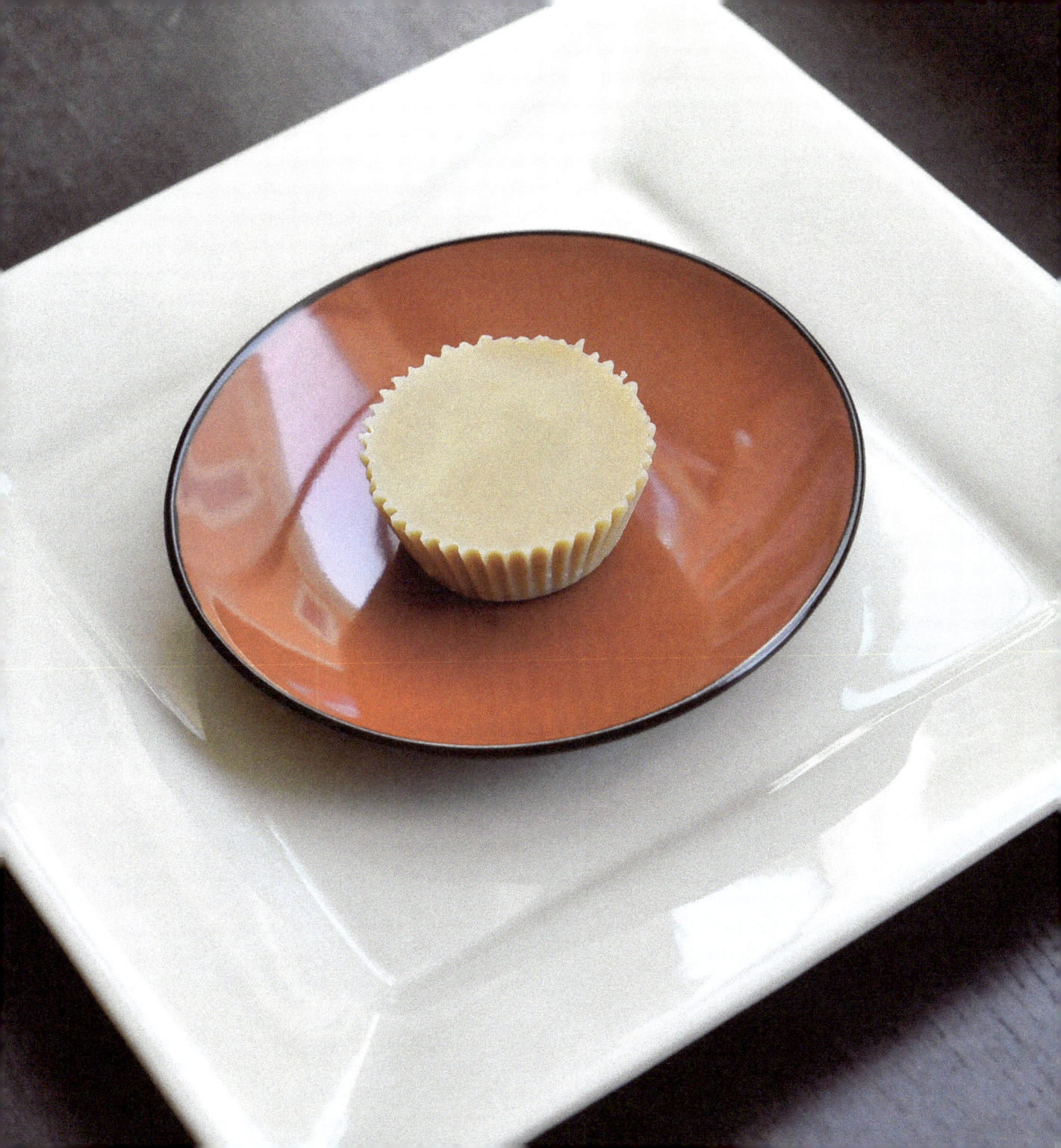

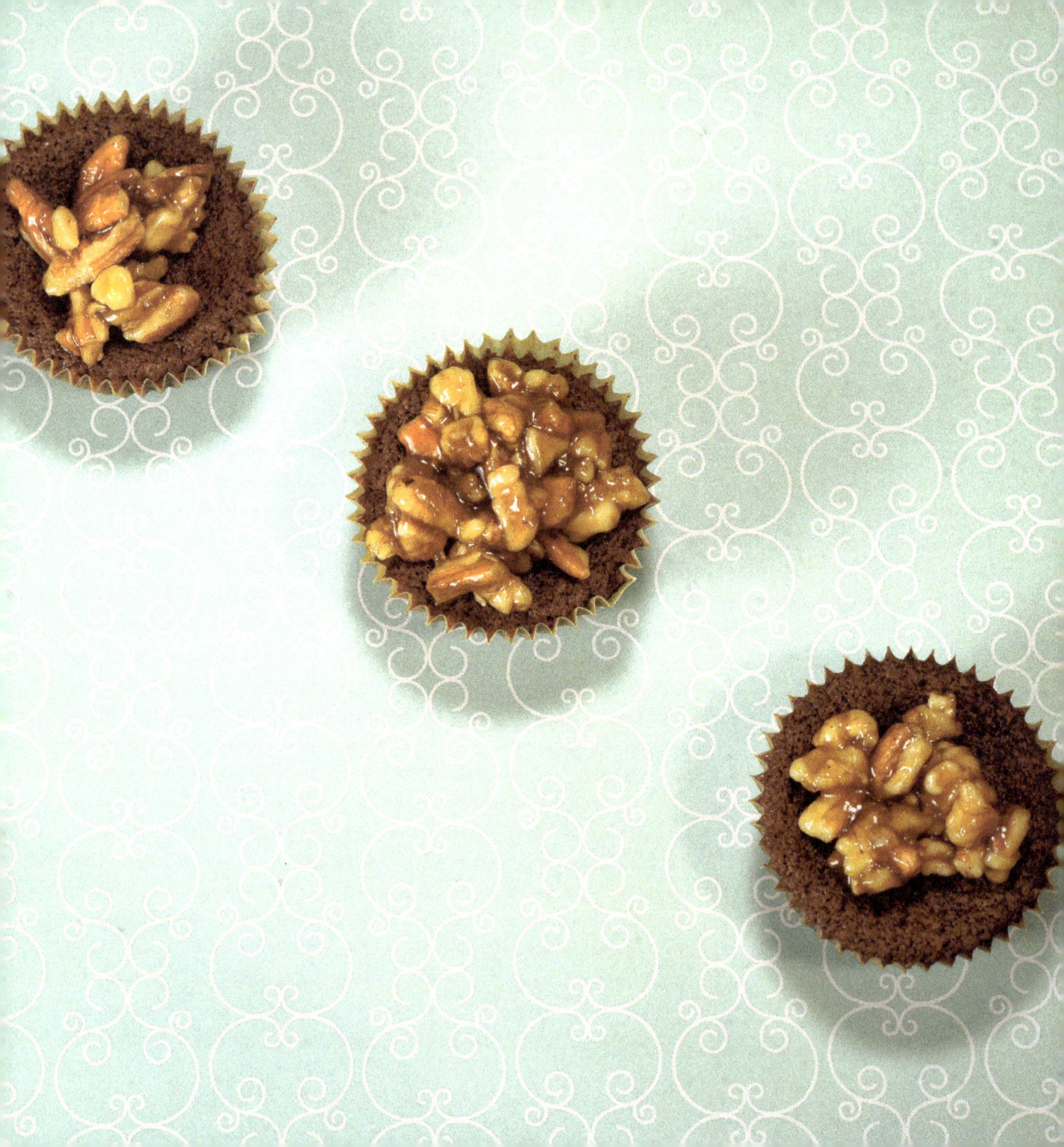

Caramel Nut Brownies
Gluten, Dairy, Egg Free
Soy & Nut Free Compatible

Soy Free Compatible: Use safe butter.
Nut Free Compatible: Use safe milk and use plain caramel sauce without nuts for garnish.

Ingredients:

Brownie Ingredients:

2 Sticks Dairy Free Butter, room temp.

2 1/2 cups Organic Sugar

3/4 cup Raw Organic Cacao Powder

2 tsp Baking Powder

1 tsp Sea Salt

1 tsp Raw Organic Ground Vanilla Bean

1 cup Organic Extra Virgin Olive Oil

6 TBSP Potato Starch

1/3 cup Organic Unsweetened Almond Milk

1 cup Water

2 cups White Sorghum Flour

Salted Nut Garnish:

1/3 cup Raw Organic Pecans

1/3 cup Raw Organic Walnuts

4 1/2 TBSP of fresh caramel sauce (page 26)

1/8 tsp Himalayan Pink Salt

Directions:

First, combine the milk and potato starch together in a glass measuring cup and set aside. Next, cream the butter and sugar together in a mixing bowl on medium speed. Add in your chocolate, salt, and vanilla, and mix again. Next, add the baking powder and milk/starch mix. Give the mix two minutes to fizz and rise. Lastly, add in your water, oil, and flour, and mix until it's all well incorporated.

Bake in a large glass dish (13x9), at 350 for 35 minutes.

As muffins, this makes 24. Bake for 24 minutes. Do not overfill the cups as the brownies will break when you try to release them, and they won't be as pretty. It's OK if the middle of the muffins sink as they cool, as it makes the perfect little "cup" for the garnish.

For the Nut Garnish
Crush the nuts, then mix them together in a bowl with the other ingredients. Scoop on top of your cooked muffins or brownie squares.

Blueberry Lemon Loaf

Gluten, Dairy, Soy, Corn Free
Paleo & GAPs Friendly

I looked forward to this treat for such a long time, and in the end, I didn't like it. Just as I was about to scrap it, the kids asked if they could try some. They all loved it, and gobbled it up, almost before I could get a good picture. That's the interesting thing about my personal story, just how much my taste buds have changed. I will say, however, the crunch top was yummy.

Ingredients:

2 Extra Large Duck Eggs (these came from a farm that specifically doesn't use corn or soy feed)

4.5 TBSP Organic Coconut Oil, room temp.

6 TBSP Organic Maple Butter

1/4 tsp Sea Salt

Juice of 2 Organic Mayer Lemons, about 4 ounces

2 TBSP Organic Black Chia Seeds

1 tsp Baking Soda

1 1/3 cup Almond Flour

1 cup Wild Organic Blueberries

4 Paper Loaf Pans 4 x 2 x 2 inch

Directions:

Start by mixing your eggs, coconut oil, maple butter, and salt together. Mix on medium-high speed to break up the coconut oil. Next, add in the lemon juice and baking soda. It will fizz a bit. Mix again on high, and the mix will foam and rise. Add in the rest of your ingredients except for the blueberries and mix on low-medium speed until it's all incorporated. Finally, fold in your blueberries and divide evenly into the four loaf pans. Alternatively, you could make muffins, but the baking time will change.

Bake at 350 for 35 minutes.

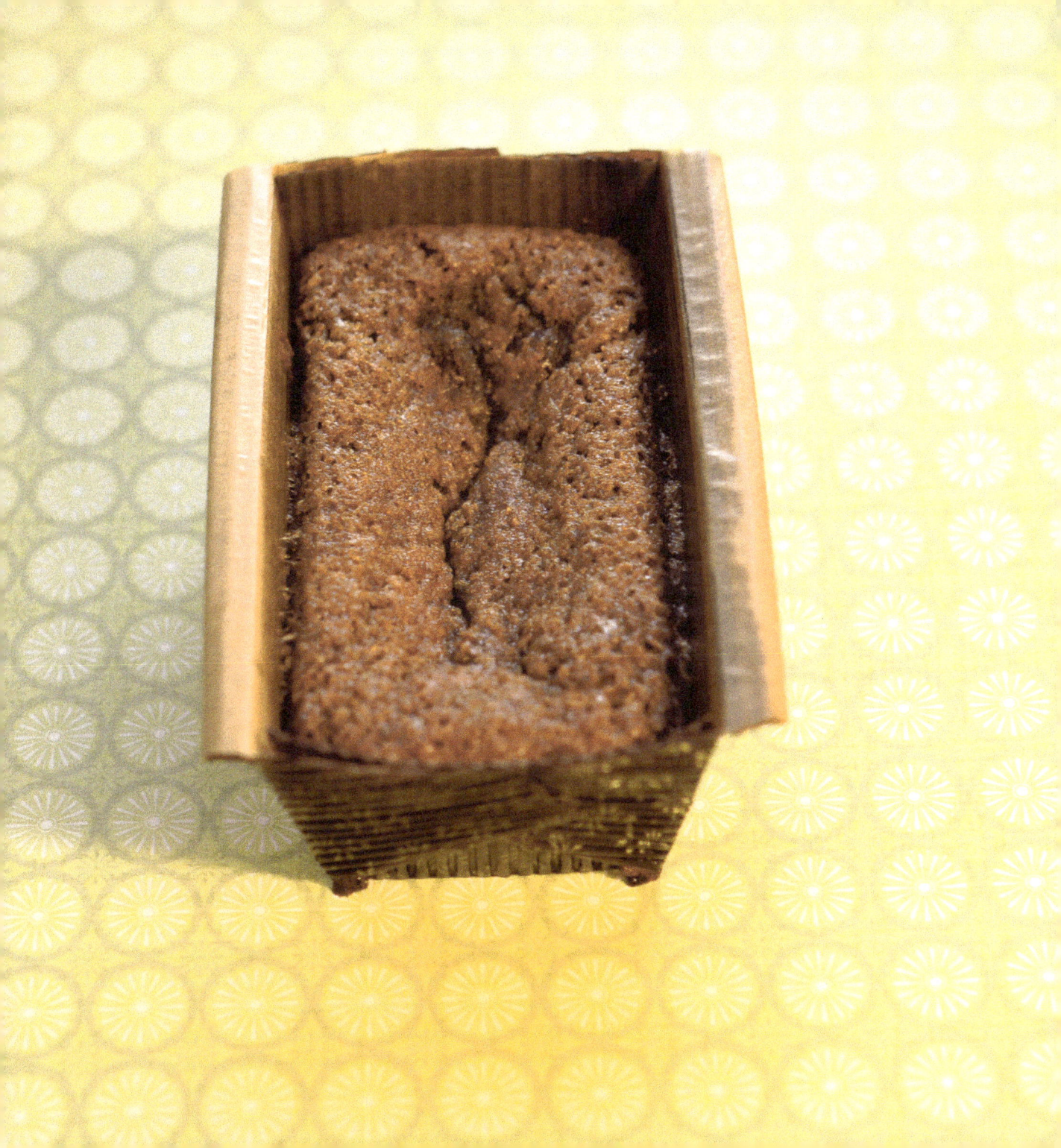

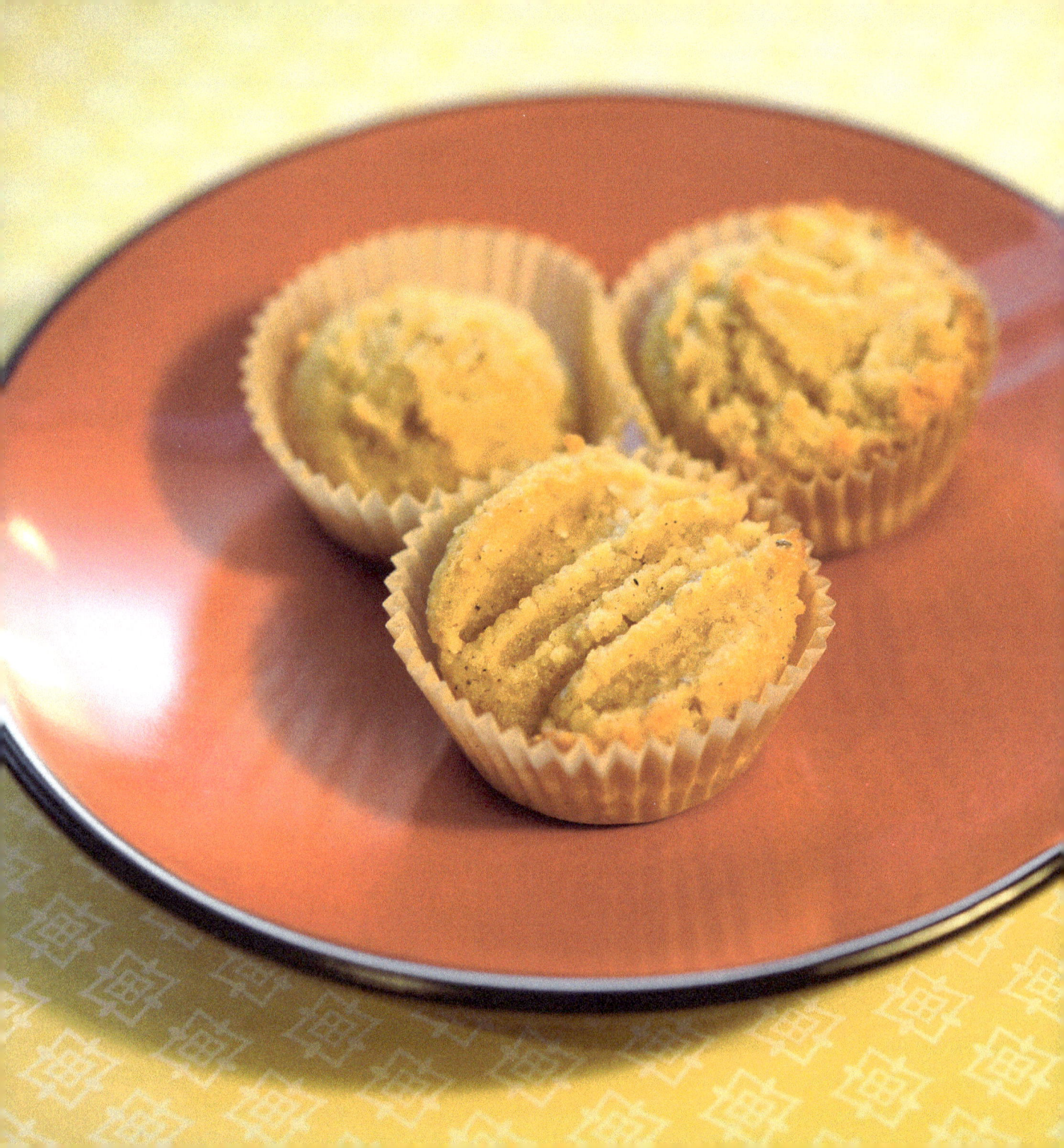

Lemon Lime Mini Muffins

Gluten, Dairy, Soy, Corn Free
Paleo & GAPs Friendly

This was inspired by the Nourish brand. I wanted to create something that was cost effective with a different flavor that I would enjoy a bit more. The little bit of lime goes a long way.

Ingredients:

2 Extra Large Duck Eggs (these came from a farm that specifically doesn't use corn or soy feed)

4.5 TBSP Organic Coconut Oil, room temp.

3 TBSP Organic Maple Butter

1/4 tsp Sea Salt

Juice of 1 Organic Mayer Lemon, about 2 ounces

Juice of 1/2 Organic Lime, I used Sweet Silver Limes

1 TBSP Organic White Chia Seeds

1/2 tsp Raw Organic Ground Vanilla Bean

1/2 tsp Baking Soda

2/3 cup Almond Flour

1/3 cup Raw Organic Coconut Flour

Directions:

Start by mixing your eggs, coconut oil, maple butter, and salt together. Mix on medium-high speed to break up the coconut oil. Next, add in the lemon juice and baking soda. Volcano! It will fizz a bit. Mix again on high, and the mix will foam and rise. Add in the rest of your ingredients and mix on low-medium speed until it's all incorporated.

I strongly suggest using a mini muffin pan for this recipe. I've found that when making Paleo items, the smaller they are, they better they cook. I used a mini muffin pan and small cookie dough scooper for these muffins.

Bake at 350 for 17 minutes.

Pumpkin Puffs

Gluten, Dairy, Egg Free
Soy & Nut Free Compatible

These were a silly thing I dreamed up one night and made them for breakfast the next day. The kids fought over who got the last one. We also served these to their friends, who simply went wild for them, and Nicolas came up with the name. This recipe also works very well with allergen ingredients: 2 eggs instead of starch/milk mix, whole milk, and wheat flour.

Soy Free Compatible: Use safe butter.
Nut Free Compatible: Use safe milk.

Ingredients:

1 Stick Dairy Free Butter, room temp.

2 Cans Organic Pumpkin Puree, nothing added

6 tsp Baking Powder

1 tsp Sea Salt

1 tsp Organic Ground Nutmeg

2 tsp Organic Ground Cinnamon

2 TBSP Organic Vanilla Extract

1/2 cup Organic Dark Brown Sugar

1 cup Enjoy Life Dark Chocolate Chips

6 TBSP Potato Starch

1 cup Organic Unsweetened Almond Milk

4C White Sorghum Flour

Mini Marshmallows, plain or pumpkin flavored (seasonal), both were a hit.

Directions:

Combine the milk and potato starch, set aside.

Next, cream the butter and sugar together in a mixing bowl on medium speed. Add in your salt, spices, and chocolate chips, and mix again. Next, add the baking powder, and milk/starch mix. Allow it to fizz and rise for 2 minutes. Lastly, add in the flour and mix until everything is incorporated.

Use an ice cream scooper or large cookie dough scooper and fill a lined muffin tray.

Bake at 350 for 10 minutes. Slide the oven rack out, keeping the tray exposed to heat, and quickly press mini marshmallows into the partially cooked batter. Close the oven and cook for another 7 minutes.

Makes 36 Puffs.

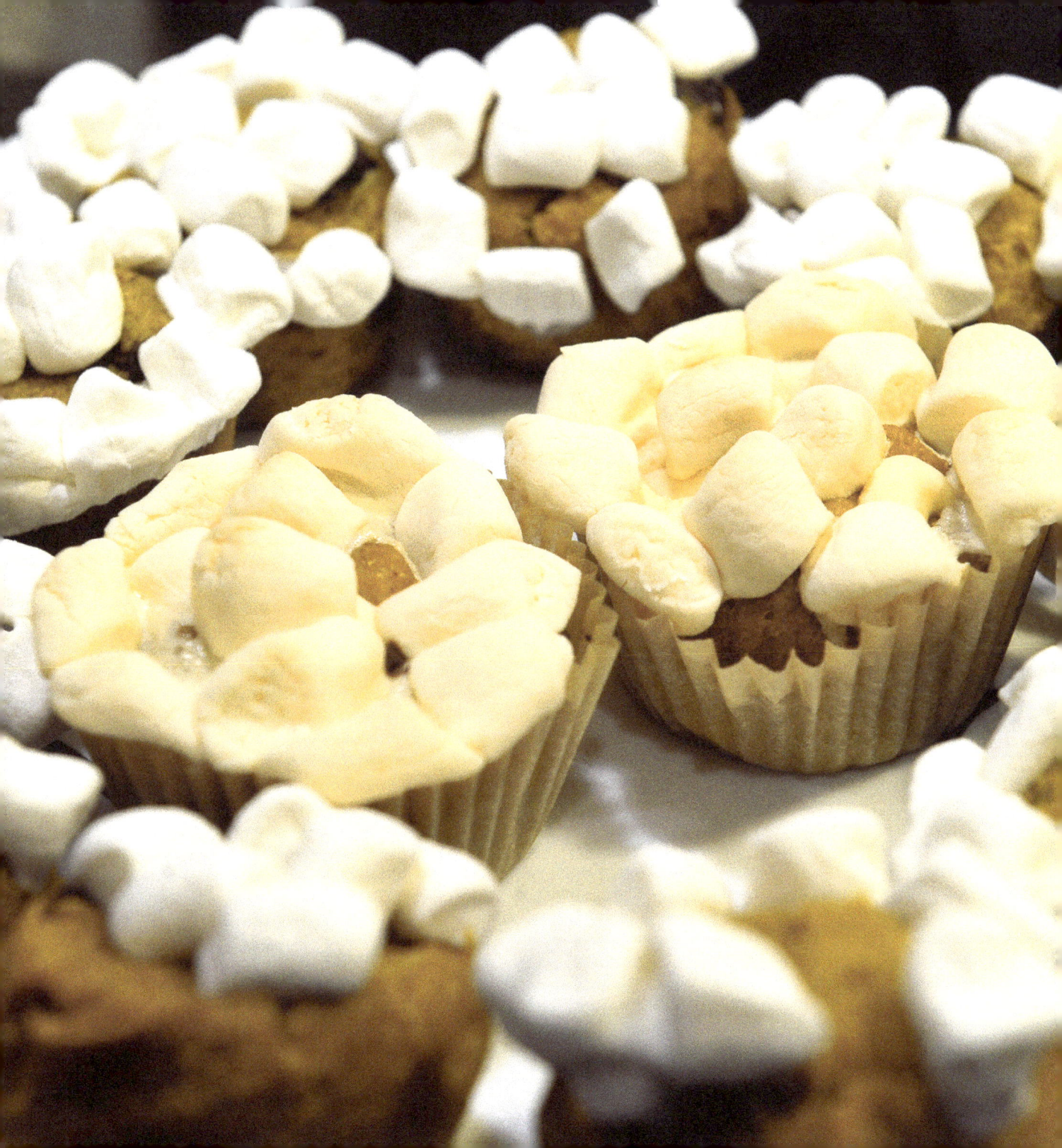

Spicy Icing
Gluten, Dairy, Egg, Nut Free
Soy Free Compatible

This is part of the cupcakes galore weekend we experienced. It was like a light went off in my head, and suddenly, there were so many new ways to top a chocolate cupcake. For the icings on the following pages, use your favorite cake mix. We've been using Pure Pantry Chocolate Cake Mix.

Soy Free Compatible: Use safe butter.

Ingredients:

1 Stick Dairy Free Butter (8T), room temp.

4 cups Organic Powdered Sugar (1 standard bag)

1/4 tsp Sea Salt

2 tsp Organic Vanilla Extract

4 TBSP Water

Organic Cayenne Pepper

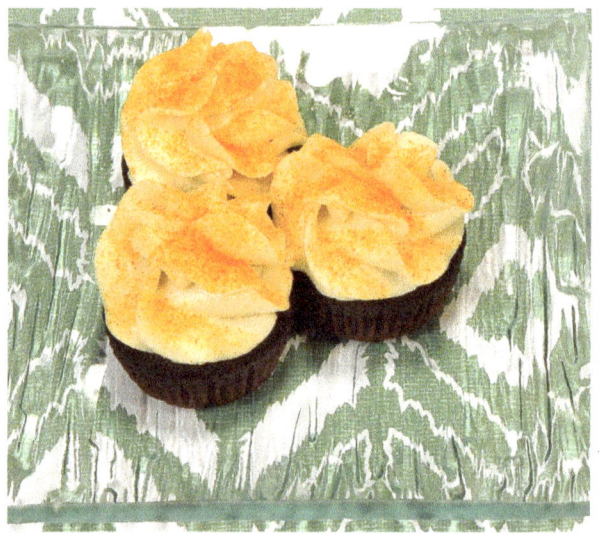

Directions:

Beat the butter on medium speed using a paddle attachment on your mixer. This will add air, creating a more fluffy icing. Add in the sugar, salt, and vanilla. One TBSP at a time, add in the water and slowly pulse. Once you have several TBSPs of water in, you should be able to mix on medium speed. Add in the last of the water. You can add up to an additional 1 TBSP of water if you want a thinner, runny, icing.

Use a tea infuser or small sieve to dust with cayenne pepper.

Ginger Icing

Gluten, Dairy, Egg, Nut Free
Soy Free Compatible

When I first thought of this one, I didn't think anyone would like it, and well, they'd think I'd lost it. I was wrong. They loved it, especially those with refined taste buds that appreciate ginger.

Soy Free Compatible: Use safe butter.

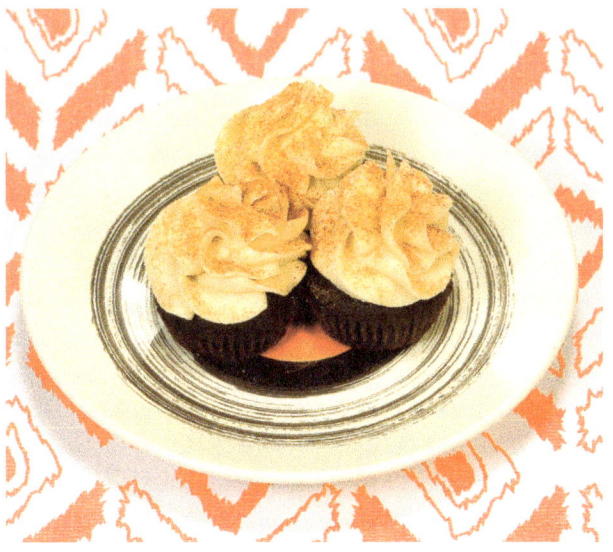

Ingredients:

1 Stick Dairy Free Butter (8T), room temp.

4 cups Organic Powdered Sugar (1 standard bag)

1/4 tsp Sea Salt

2 tsp Organic Vanilla Extract

4 TBSP Water

Organic Ground Ginger

Organic Ground Cinnamon

Directions:

Beat the butter on medium speed using a paddle attachment on your mixer. This will add air, creating a more fluffy icing. Add in the sugar, salt, and vanilla. One TBSP at a time, add in the water and slowly pulse. Once you have several TBSPs of water in, you should be able to mix on medium speed. Add in the last of the water. You can add up to another 1 TBSP of water if you want a thinner, runny, icing.

Use a tea infuser or small sieve for dusting. Do a little ginger on the first pass, and then cinnamon on the second pass. I aimed for a 1:2 ratio.

Graham Cracker Crunch Icing

Gluten, Dairy, Egg, Nut Free

During the now famous cupcake weekend, I knew not everything could be the same. I realized it would be great to have a silky, creamy, chocolaty icing... funny thing is, I hate chocolate. I do however love the idea of a hint of chocolate, hence, this icing was born. The crunch just makes it that much better.

Ingredients:

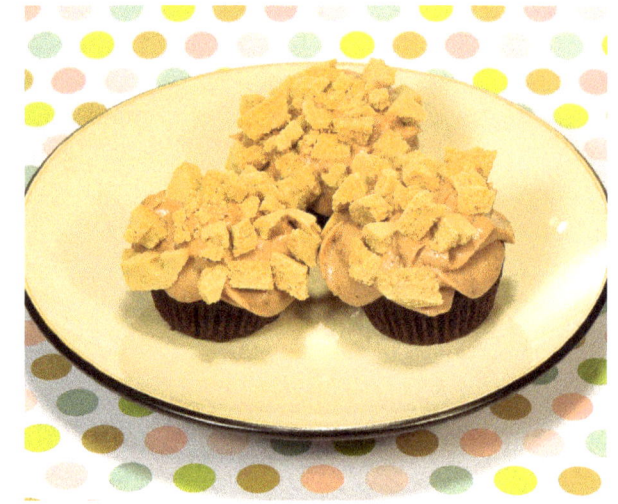

1 Stick Dairy Free Butter (8T), room temp.

8 ounces Dairy Free Cream Cheese

4 cups Organic Powdered Sugar (1 standard bag)

1/4 cup Raw Organic Cacao Powder

1/4 tsp Sea Salt

2 tsp Organic Vanilla Extract

4 TBSP water

Graham Crackers, GF DF EF, Kinnikinnick brand

Directions:

Beat the butter and cream cheese together on medium speed using a paddle attachment on your mixer. This will add air, creating a more fluffy icing. Add in all of the other ingredients, except the water, and pulse together. Add in the water 1 TBSP at a time and mix on low-medium speed until it's well incorporated. Don't over mix.

Use a large sharp knife to cut the graham crackers into small pieces. If you're OK with crumbs, use a mallet, but we opted to cut to control the size. Top the cupcakes with icing, and gently roll through the graham crackers. You may need to place a few more on by hand.

Creme Cookie Crunch Cupcakes & Icing

Gluten, Dairy, Egg, Nut Free

These were a H-I-T! I can't tell you how much these were loved by all types of eaters. These can be made as minis with the topping only, or as a standard cupcake with a cookie in the middle.

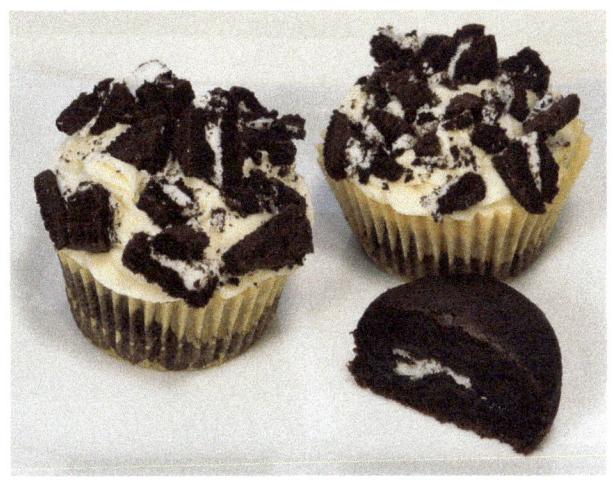

Ingredients:

1 Stick Dairy Free Butter (8T), room temp.

4 cups Organic Powdered Sugar (1 standard bag)

1/4 tsp Sea Salt

2 tsp Organic Vanilla Extract

4 TBSP water

Creme Cookies GF DF EF, Kinnikinnick brand

Directions:

For a cookie filled cupcake, fill your liner with cake batter half way, place in a whole cookie flat, then cover with more batter. Bake the cake as normal. No time or temperature changes are needed.

Beat the butter on medium speed using a paddle attachment on your mixer. This will add air, creating a more fluffy icing. Add in the sugar, salt, and vanilla. One TBSP at a time, add in the water and slowly pulse. After 3 TBSPs of water, you should be able to mix on medium speed. Add in the last of the water and continue to mix.

Use a large sharp knife to cut the cookies into small pieces to control the size. Top the cupcakes with icing, and gently roll through the cookies. You may need to place a few more on by hand.

Cream Filled Strawberry Cupcake

Gluten, Dairy, Egg, Nut Free
Soy Free Compatible

Filled cupcakes are simply a joy. It's that little surprise you weren't expecting. In the past, I wasn't able to create something like this as all of the dairy free cream options weren't viable. However, So Delicious has done it again. They now make a wonderful coconut whip that you can find in the freezer section.

Soy Free Compatible: Use safe butter.

Ingredients:

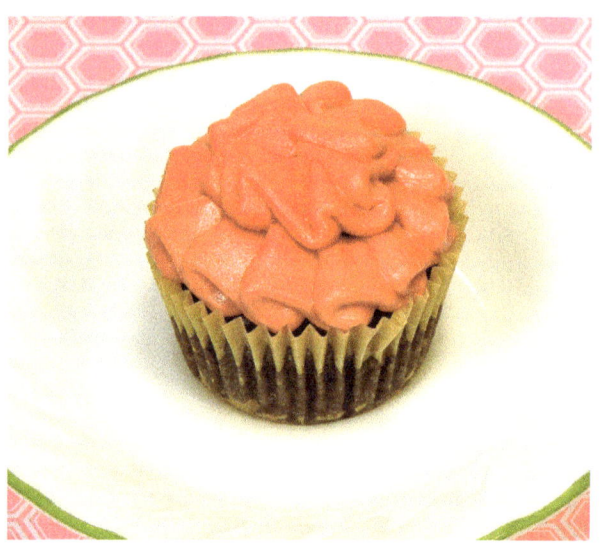

1 Stick Dairy Free Butter (8T), room temp.

4 cups Organic Powdered Sugar (1 standard bag)

1/4 tsp Sea Salt

2 tsp Organic Vanilla Extract

1 tsp Strawberry Flavoring

4 TBSP water

Natural Red Coloring, India Tree brand

Organic Coconut Whip, So Delicious brand, freezer item (or your preferred cream)

Directions:

To fill the cupcake, place a Bismarck Tip into a decorator bag. Once the whip is thawed, place several scoops into your bag and gently fill. I fill each cupcake in 3 different spots to ensure maximum fill.

To make the icing, beat the butter on medium speed using a paddle attachment on your mixer. This will add air, creating a more fluffy icing. Add in the sugar, salt, strawberry, and vanilla. One TBSP at a time, add in the water and slowly pulse. Add in as much red as you'd like to reach the desired tint. Mix until it's all incorporated and a fluffy icing has formed.

Peppermint Icing

Gluten, Dairy, Egg, Nut Free
Soy Free Compatible

For years, this has been a crowd favorite among those that eat our food. To enhance the flavor, during Christmas time we top with organic crushed candy cane.

Soy Free Compatible: Use safe butter.

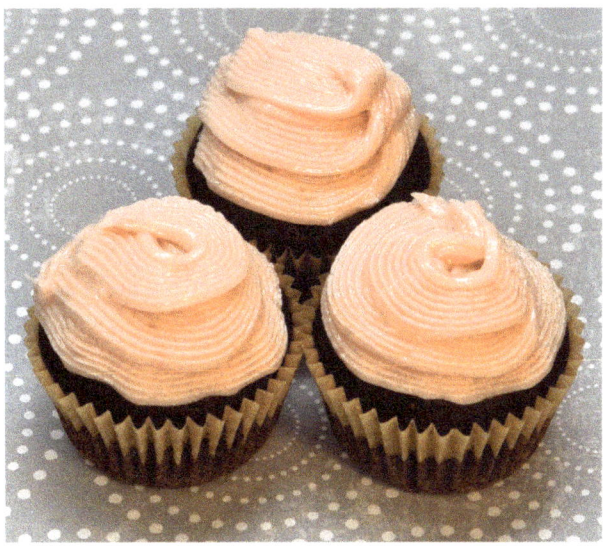

Ingredients:

1 Stick Dairy Free Butter (8T), room temp.

4 cups Organic Powdered Sugar (1 standard bag)

1/4 tsp Sea Salt

2 tsp Organic Vanilla Extract

1 tsp Organic Peppermint Extract

4 TBSP Water

10 Drops Red Food Coloring, India Tree brand, use more for a more intense red.

Directions:

Beat the butter on medium speed using a paddle attachment on your mixer. This will add air, creating a more fluffy icing. Add in the sugar, salt, peppermint, and vanilla. One TBSP at a time, add in the water and slowly pulse. Once you have 3 TBSPs of water in, you should be able to mix on medium speed. Add in the last of the water, and the red drops.

Banana Cream Cheese Icing

Gluten, Dairy, Egg, Nut Free
Soy Free Compatible

There were three versions of this icing, but the one below is the one that everyone consistently said was the best. The other variations used freeze dried bananas instead of fresh. The caveat is that this icing is runny by nature. If you'd prefer a thicker icing, crush freeze dried banana and use in place of the fresh.

Soy Free Compatible: Use safe butter.

Ingredients:

1 Stick Dairy Free Butter (8T), room temp.

4 ounces Dairy Free Cream Cheese

6 cups Organic Powdered Sugar (1.5 standard bag)

1/4 cup Organic Light Brown Sugar, packed

1/4 tsp Sea Salt

2 tsp Organic Vanilla Extract

1.5 Large Organic Banana, mushed with a fork

1 cup Tapioca Starch

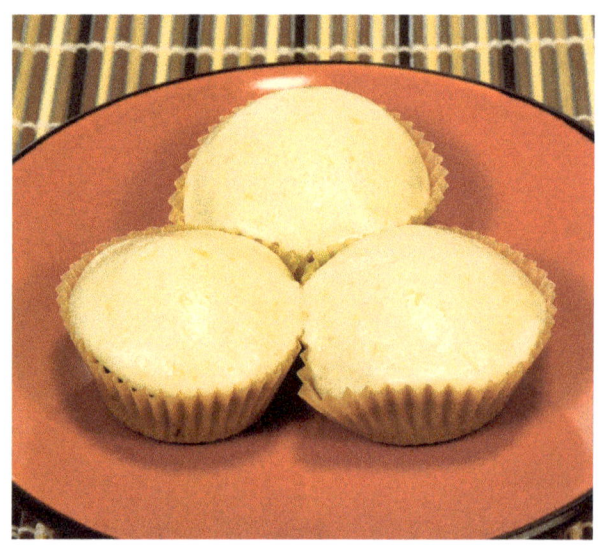

Directions:

Beat the butter and cream cheese together on medium speed using a paddle attachment on your mixer. This will add air, creating a more fluffy icing. Scrape down the edges of the bowl and mix again. Add in the rest of your ingredients and mix again; it comes together quickly.

If you try the freeze dried bananas, use a Vitamix Dry Container to crush the bananas and brown sugar together. We experimented with a 2.5 ounce bag of freeze dried banana.

Peanut Butter Icing

Gluten, Dairy, Egg Free
Soy & Corn Free Compatible

Soy Free Compatible: Use safe butter.
Corn Free Compatible: Source safe ingredients. Start with a safe butter, or butter replacement. Be sure your powdered sugar doesn't have corn starch, such as the 365 brand which uses potato starch. If you don't have access to safe peanut butter, you could try almond butter. For the vanilla extract, make your own using potato vodka, or use ground vanilla bean.

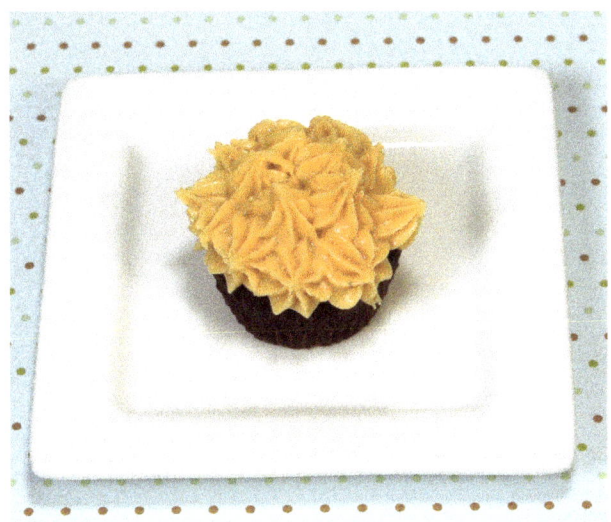

Ingredients:

1 Stick Dairy Free Butter (8T), room temp.

9 TBSP Organic Creamy Peanut Butter

4 cups Organic Powdered Sugar (1 standard bag)

1/2 tsp Sea Salt

3 tsp Organic Vanilla Extract

7 TBSP water

Directions:

Using a paddle attachment on your mixer, combine the butter and peanut butter on medium speed. Next, add in the other ingredients, excluding the water. Pulse together, then add in the water 1 TBSP at a time. Continue to pulse until you're able to leave the mixer on medium speed without making a mess. Mix until a nice icing forms.

Cashew Chocolate Smoothie

Gluten, Dairy, Egg, Soy Free
Paleo Friendly, Corn Free Compatible

I am a firm believer in the institution of ice cream. When we first purchased our Vitamix, it was because I was overworking our low powered blender. It started with "normal" smoothies until I accidentally discovered the proper combination of frozen ingredients mimic ice cream. We've never looked back.

Corn Free Compatible: Use option 1, and source safe ingredients.

Option 1:

1.5 cup Raw Organic Cashews

1/3 cup Raw Organic Cacao Powder

4 TBSP Raw Organic Honey

1 TBSP Organic Vanilla Extract
(1 tsp ground vanilla bean for Paleo)

1/2 tsp Organic Peppermint Extract

3/4 cup Water

2.5 cups Ice

Option 2:

4 Organic Bananas

2 cups Raw Organic Cashews

1/3c Raw Organic Cacao Powder

3 TBSP Raw Organic Honey

1/2 tsp Organic Peppermint Extract

1/3 cup Water

1.5 cups Ice

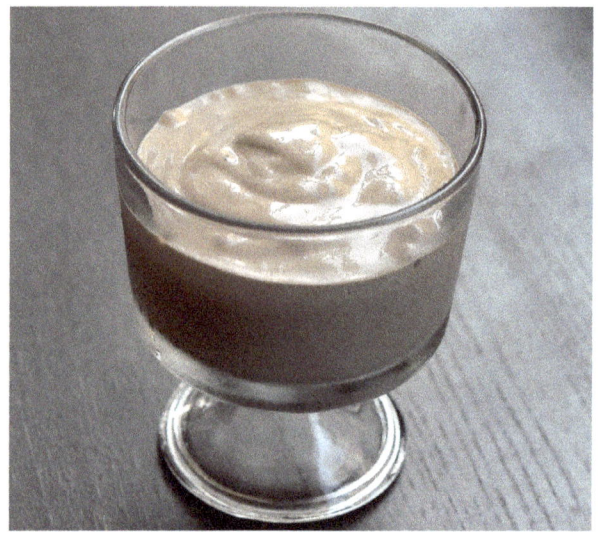

Directions:

Mix everything but the ice to create a smooth base. Add the ice and mix again. Try not to over mix the base which creates heat. More heat means more ice to achieve the milkshake texture. Too much ice can create a watery flavor.

Spinach Blueberry Smoothie

Gluten, Dairy, Egg, Soy Free
Paleo & GAPs Friendly

When I created this, I really thought the kids would hate it. To my surprise, the younger two exclaimed that it tasted like candy and asked for seconds. I hope this healthy drink is a hit in your home too.

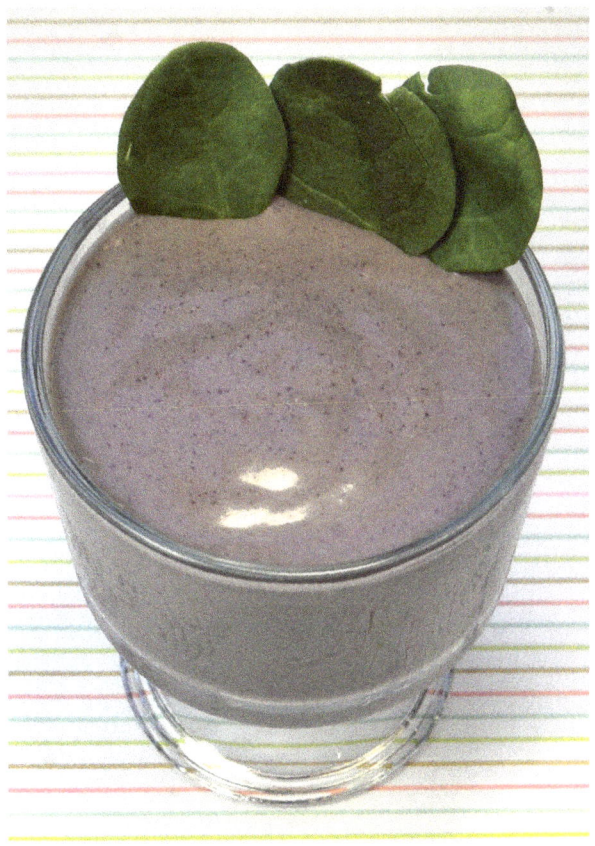

Ingredients:

1.5 cup Raw Organic Cashews

3 Large Organic Bananas

10 ounces Wild Organic Blueberries, frozen

1 cup Compressed Organic Spinach

4.5 TBSP Raw Organic Honey

1 cup Water

2.5 cups Ice

Directions:

To measure the spinach, press down on it as you add it to the measuring cup. By removing the air, you're getting a more accurate cup of spinach. Mix everything but the ice to create a smooth base. Add the ice and mix again.

Strawberry Cashew Smoothie

Gluten, Dairy, Egg, Soy Free
Paleo & GAPs Friendly

This drink has become another "candy" that the kids request. It makes for a great addition to breakfast, or as an after school snack.

Ingredients:

2 cups Raw Organic Cashews

2 tsp Organic Vanilla Extract
(1 tsp Ground Vanilla for Paleo & GAPs)

2 Large Organic Bananas

20 ounces Organic Whole Frozen Strawberries

1/2 cup Organic Maple Syrup

1 cup Water

Ice is optional if you'd like a different texture or need to have an extra serving.

Directions:

Blend everything but the ice together in a Vitamix or high powered blender until smooth. Mix again if you choose to add ice.

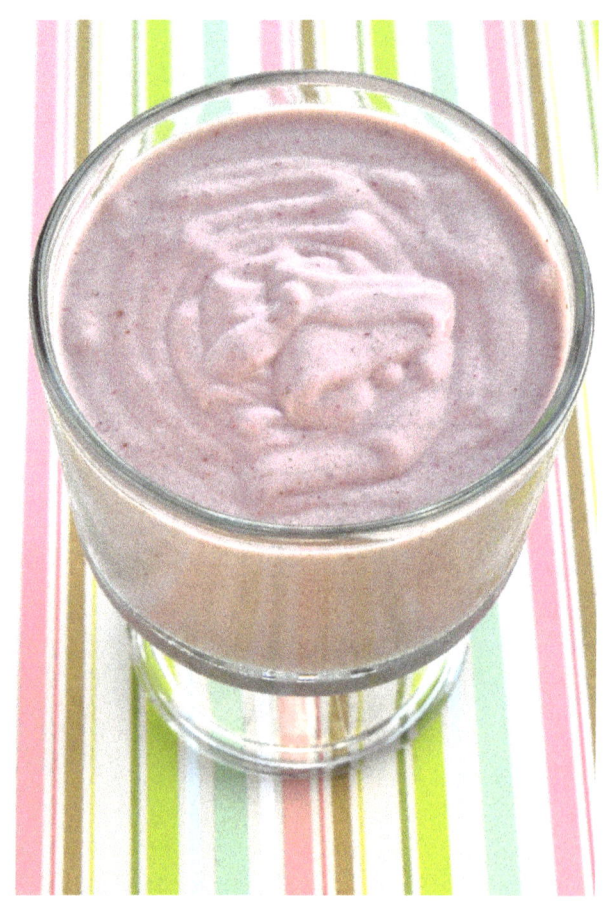

Tropical "Ice Cream" in Passion Fruit Cup & Lemonade Cream Sauce

Gluten, Dairy, Egg, Nut, Soy Free
Paleo & GAPs Friendly

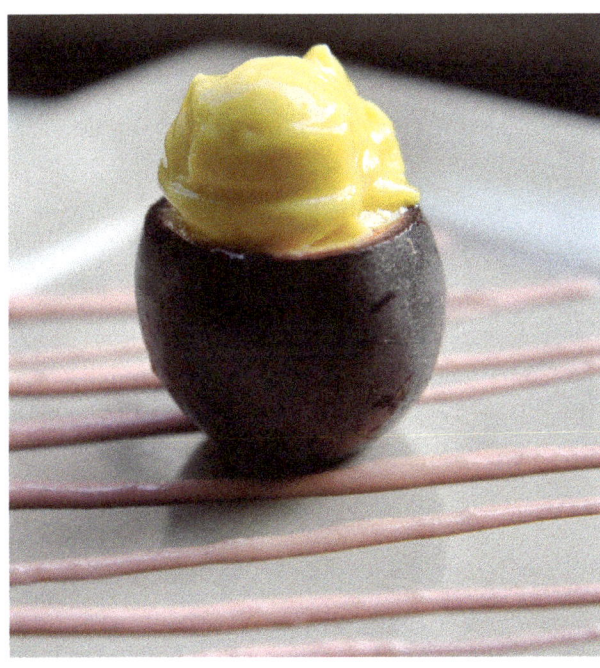

Ingredients:

Ice Cream:

10 Ounces Organic Frozen Pineapple

10 Ounces Organic Frozen Mango

2/3 cup Organic Milk of choice

1/3 cup Organic Maple Syrup

Passion Fruit

Sauce:

14 Organic Strawberries, fresh and hulled

2 ounces Organic Lemon Juice

10 ounces Whip of choice, we've used both Soyatoo and So Delicious Coconut Whip

Directions:

In a blender, blend your sauce ingredients together and set aside. Place the sauce in a squeeze bottle if you'd like a fancy plating. Next, carefully cut the top off your passion fruit and gently remove and discard the insides. A grapefruit spoon works really well. Also cut a tiny bit off the bottom so it will stand. Finally, blend the ice cream ingredients together, and spoon into your passion fruit cup.

Paleo Fruit Pastry

Gluten, Dairy, Egg, Soy, Corn Free
Paleo & GAPs Friendly

After months of pondering how to create this, and finding safe ingredients, I present my little victory.

Ingredients:

1/2 cup Coconut Flour, raw OK

4.5 TBSP Organic Coconut Oil, room temp.

1 TBSP Organic Maple Butter

1/4 tsp Sea Salt

1 cup Blanched Almond Meal

4 TBSP Water

1 Large Organic Apple, blended

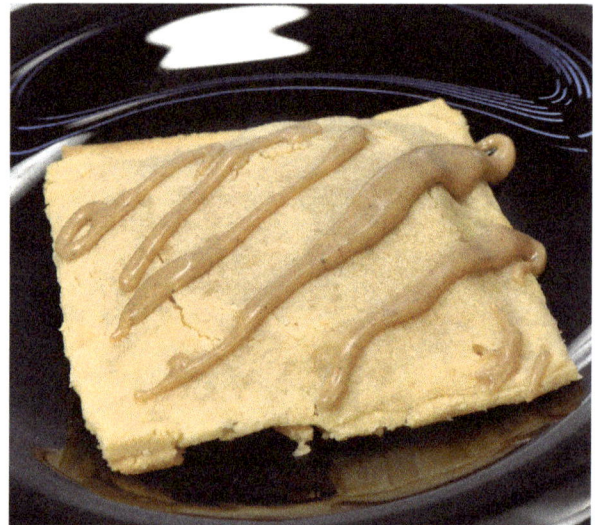

Glaze:

2 tsp Organic Maple Butter

4 dashes of Raw Organic Ground Vanilla Bean

2 dashes of Organic Cinnamon & nutmeg, optional

Directions:

Mix your dough ingredients until a dough forms. Place in a gallon sized baggie and press flat. Chill in the fridge for at least 1 hour. Roll flat on parchment paper and cut into squares. Place a spoonful of blended apple on a square and top with another. Carefully pinch the edges together, the dough is delicate. Bake at 350 for 8 minutes. To make the glaze, whisk the ingredients together in a small bowl.

Jam Filled Pastry

Gluten, Dairy, Egg, Nut Free
Soy Free Compatible

A long time ago, before we knew that Kid Two had a wheat issue, we would make homemade jam pastries. Needless to say, as allergies crop up, one must start to think outside the box. All of the kids have told me how great these taste. Hopefully you'll have similar results.

Soy Free Compatible: Use safe butter.

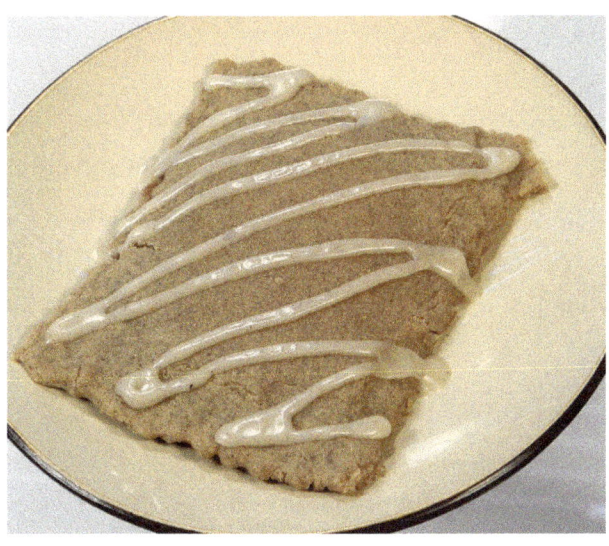

Ingredients:

1 Stick Dairy Free Butter (8T), room temp.

1 1/2 cup White Sorghum Flour

6 TBSP Water

3 TBSP Potato Starch

1/4 tsp Sea Salt

Jam, Fruit Spread, or Preserves of choice

We made a simple glaze with powdered sugar, ground vanilla bean, cinnamon, nutmeg, and almond milk.

Directions:

Mix your dough ingredients until a dough forms. Place in a gallon sized baggie and press flat. Chill in the fridge for at least 1 hour. Roll flat on parchment paper and cut into squares. Place 1 TBSP of jam on a square and cover with another square. Pinch the edges together with a fork.

Bake at 350 for 10 minutes. Allow these to cool a bit before adding glaze to prevent the glaze from melting.

Stuffed Apple Cups

Gluten, Dairy, Egg, Soy Free
Optionally Nut Free, Paleo & GAPs Friendly, Corn Free Compatible

Corn Free Compatible: Source safe ingredients.

Who doesn't like apple pie, right? I still giggle a little to myself as I remember the first time we made these. The kids tried to eat them hot, right out of the oven.

Ingredients:

3 Large Organic Fuji Apples

1 Small Organic Apple, your favorite kind

15 Organic Brazil Nuts, crushed

1 cup of apple blend (below)

Apple Blend

20 ounces (weight) of Organic Cubed Apple

1/3 cup Organic Maple Syrup

1/4 tsp Raw Organic Ground Vanilla

3/4 tsp Organic Ground Cinnamon

1/8 tsp Ground Organic Nutmeg

1 dash of Organic Ground Cloves

There will be extra blend left over. I like to put it in the kids' lunches as a nice treat.

Directions:

First, make your apple blend. Place all of the ingredients in your blender, and start by mixing on low speed. This will make an apple liquid on the bottom, and then you can turn your blender up to a higher speed and it will blend easier.

Cut off the top of the apple, 1/4 to 1/2 an inch. Next, use a melon baller to core out the three large apples. Leave a border of apple as you core it. It's best to twist the melon baller all the way around to prevent tearing the apple away.

Finally, combine the crushed nuts with 1 cup of the apple blend, and spoon into your apple cups. Bake at 350 for 30 minutes.

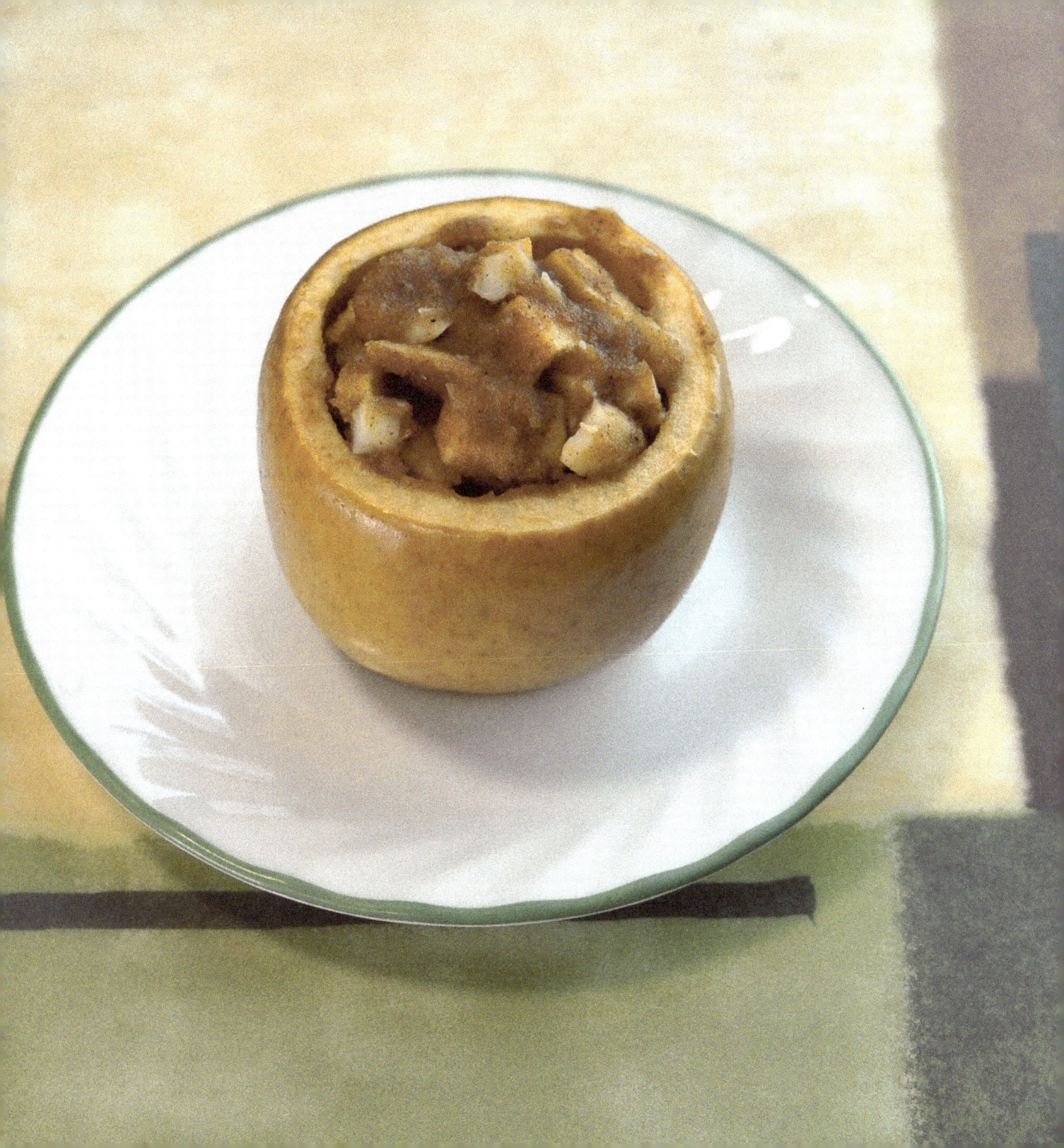

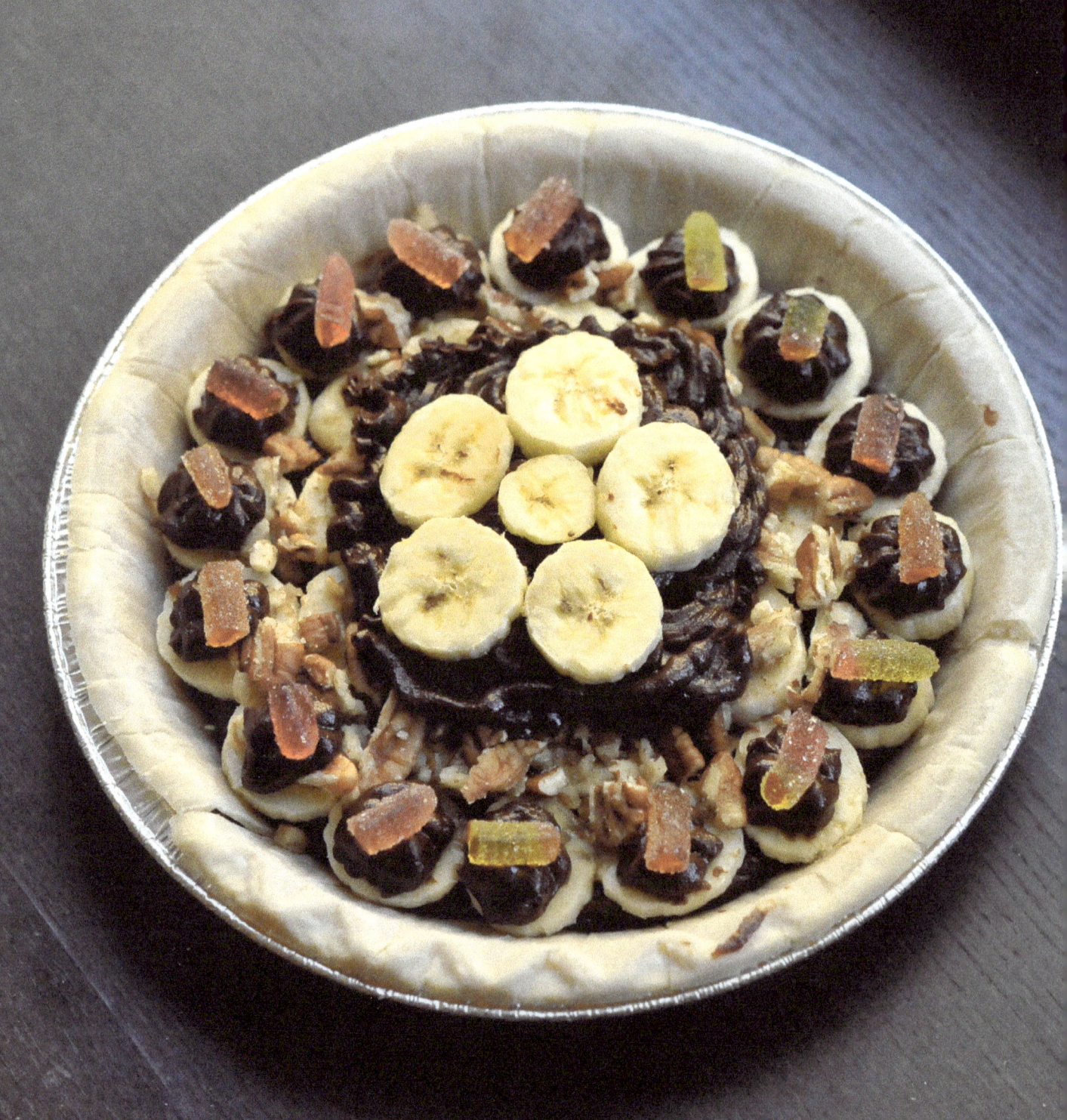

Fudgey Banana Date Pie

Gluten, Dairy, Egg, Soy Free
Optionally Nut Free, Paleo Compatible

Nut Free: Omit the pecan garnish.
Paleo Compatible: Omit the GF pie crust and use a nut crust, or no crust at all.

Ingredients:

1 Wholly Wholesome GF Pie Crust
(rice based, sold in the freezer section)

3-4 Organic Bananas, depending on size and
thickness of your slices

1/2 cup Organic Pecans, smashed into pieces

4 Organic Sour Worms, optional

Fudge Filling:

20 Organic Medjool Dates, medium to large in
size. The juicer, the better.

1/3 cup Raw Organic Cacao Powder

1/2 cup Organic Unsweetened Almond Milk

A little back-story for you... I reached a point
one day where I hated that Kid Three always had
to have a lot less than the next guy. I started my
mission to create a GF, DF, EF, Low sugar dessert
that everyone could eat. The look of shock on his
face when he got a normal slice was worth the
hard work. I encourage you to use this as a spring
board for your own creations.

Directions:

Bake your pie crust in the oven for 10 minutes,
and set aside to cool.

Remove the pits from the dates, combine with
chocolate and milk in your blender. It's OK if it
warms up in the process. Set aside when done.

Slice your worms and bananas, and get ready to
assemble.

Spread 1/4 - 1/3 of your chocolate mix in the
bottom of the pie crust. This provides the "glue"
to hold things together. Layer in bananas and
get as many to fit as you can. Carefully spread
in 3/4 of the remaining chocolate on top of the
bananas. Make sure to get into all the little cracks,
and go all the way to the edges. Add another
layer of bananas. Sprinkle the pecans all over the
center. Put the remainder of your chocolate in a
decorating bag and dot the outer bananas with
chocolate. Add a small center layer of chocolate
and banana. Last, add the worms.

Refrigerate for at least 2 hours, and serve cold.

Now Entering The Doughnut Zone

All of the doughnut recipes were all made using a mini doughnut maker. You can purchase one online such as the Babycakes or Bella Cucina brands. We used non-stick spray for each batch as well, which is very important to ensure the doughnuts come out properly. I have seen baking trays that are mini doughnut molds, but we haven't tested these. I would be wary of something like that given the release issues with GF DF EF baking we've encountered.

Tools you will need:
- Doughnut Maker
- Decorating Bags
- Decorating Tips
- Skewers

If you decide to make several variations at once, save time by making only one batch of vanilla icing and then dividing it into equal parts before adding flavors and colors. Each of these recipes provides a quarter batch of icing.

If you add color to your icing, be careful, as the extra liquid can cause the icing to become runny. Try to plan ahead and make the icing thicker by using less water. Also be aware that if you use natural colors, such as India Tree, the color "fades" and "runs" over night.

I found that 3 minutes in the doughnut maker was a good amount of time. I then cooled them by "hanging" them on a skewer over a bowl.

Allow the doughnuts to cool before icing. Serve fresh. These have a short shelf life of less than 36 hours.

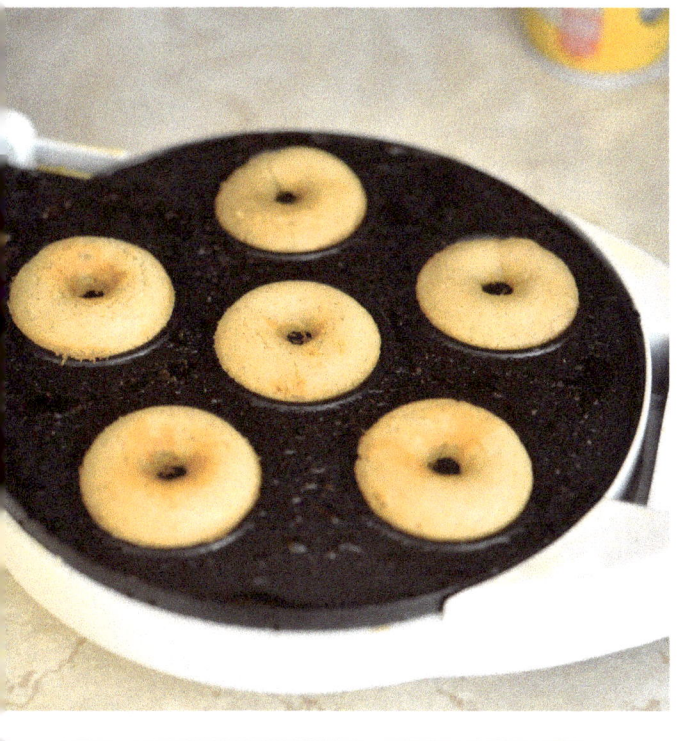
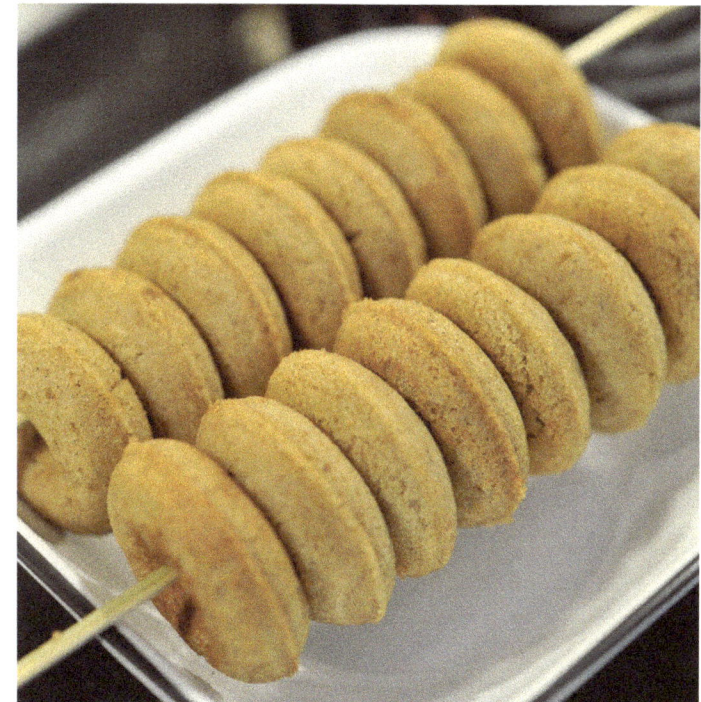
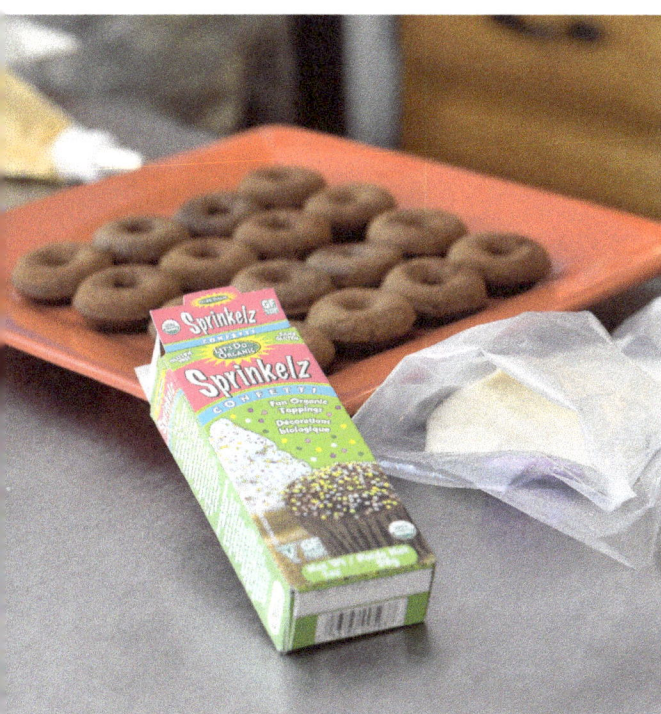
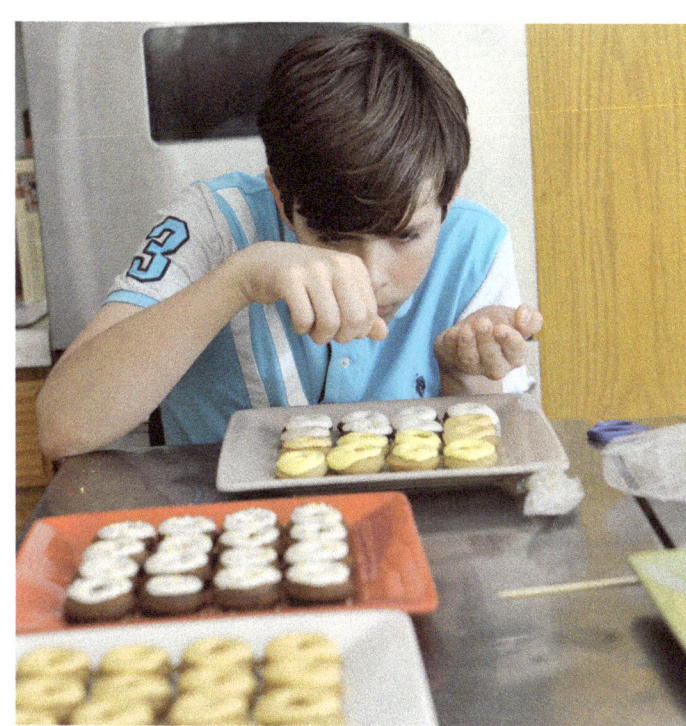

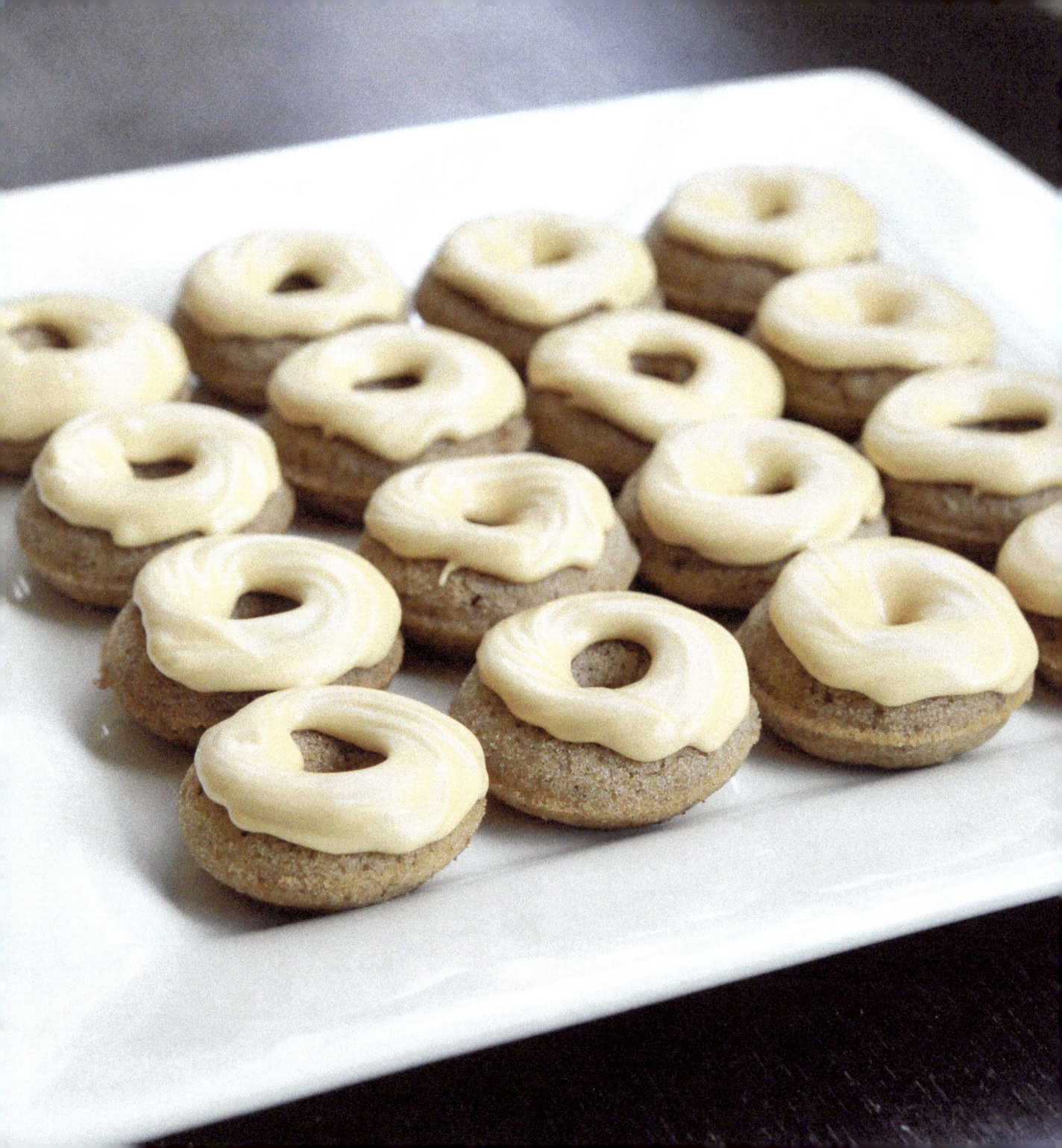

Cinnamon Doughnut with Orange Icing

Gluten, Dairy, Egg Free
Nut & Soy Free Compatible

Nut Free: Use safe milk.
Soy Free: Use safe butter.

Ingredients:

3 TBSP Dairy Free Butter

1/4 cup Organic Sugar

1 TBSP Potato Starch

1 tsp Baking Powder

Dash of Sea Salt

1/2 cup + 1 TBSP Milk,
we used Unsweetened Almond Milk

3/4 cup White Sorghum Flour

1 tsp Organic Vanilla Extract

1 tsp Organic Ground Cinnamon

1/2 tsp Organic Ground Nutmeg

Icing:

2 TBSP Dairy Free Butter, room temp.

1 cup Organic Powdered Sugar

Dash of Sea Salt

1/8 tsp Organic Orange Extract/Flavoring

1 TBSP Water

Directions:

Review the notes on page 64 before starting.

Using the wire attachment on your mixer, combine the doughnut ingredients on medium speed. Once everything is incorporated, place batter into a decorating bag. This will help ensure accurate placement of the batter.

Cut the tip off of the decorating bag and pipe the batter into your (pre-heated) doughnut maker. I found that 3 minutes in the doughnut maker was a good amount of time.

Allow the doughnuts to cool by "hanging" them on a skewer over a bowl before icing. If you add color to your icing, be careful, as the extra liquid can cause the icing to become runny. Try to plan ahead and make the icing thicker by using less water.

Note: Unlike the other three doughnut recipes, these have an even shorter shelf life of less than 24 hours. This particular variation becomes more dry, faster.

Chocolate Doughnut

Gluten, Dairy, Egg, Nut Free
Nut & Soy Free Compatible

Nut Free: Use safe milk.
Soy Free: Use safe butter.

Ingredients:

3 TBSP Dairy Free Butter

1/4 + 1/8 cup Organic Sugar

1 TBSP Potato Starch

1 tsp Baking Powder

Dash of Sea Salt

1/2 cup Organic Unsweetened Almond Milk

1/2 + 1/8 cup White Sorghum Flour

1/4 cup Buckwheat Flour

1/4 cup Raw Organic Cocoa Powder

Icing:

2 TBSP Dairy Free Butter, room temp.

1 cup Organic Powdered Sugar

Dash of Sea Salt

1/2 tsp Organic Vanilla Extract

1 TBSP Water

1/8 tsp Organic Peppermint Extract

Directions:

Review the notes on page 64 before starting.

Using the wire attachment on your mixer, combine the doughnut ingredients on medium speed. Once everything is incorporated, place batter into a decorating bag. This will help ensure accurate placement of the batter.

Cut the tip off of the decorating bag and pipe the batter into your (pre-heated) doughnut maker. I found that 3 minutes in the doughnut maker was a good amount of time.

Allow the doughnuts to cool by "hanging" them on a skewer over a bowl before icing. These have a short shelf life of less than 36 hours, so it's best to serve them fresh.

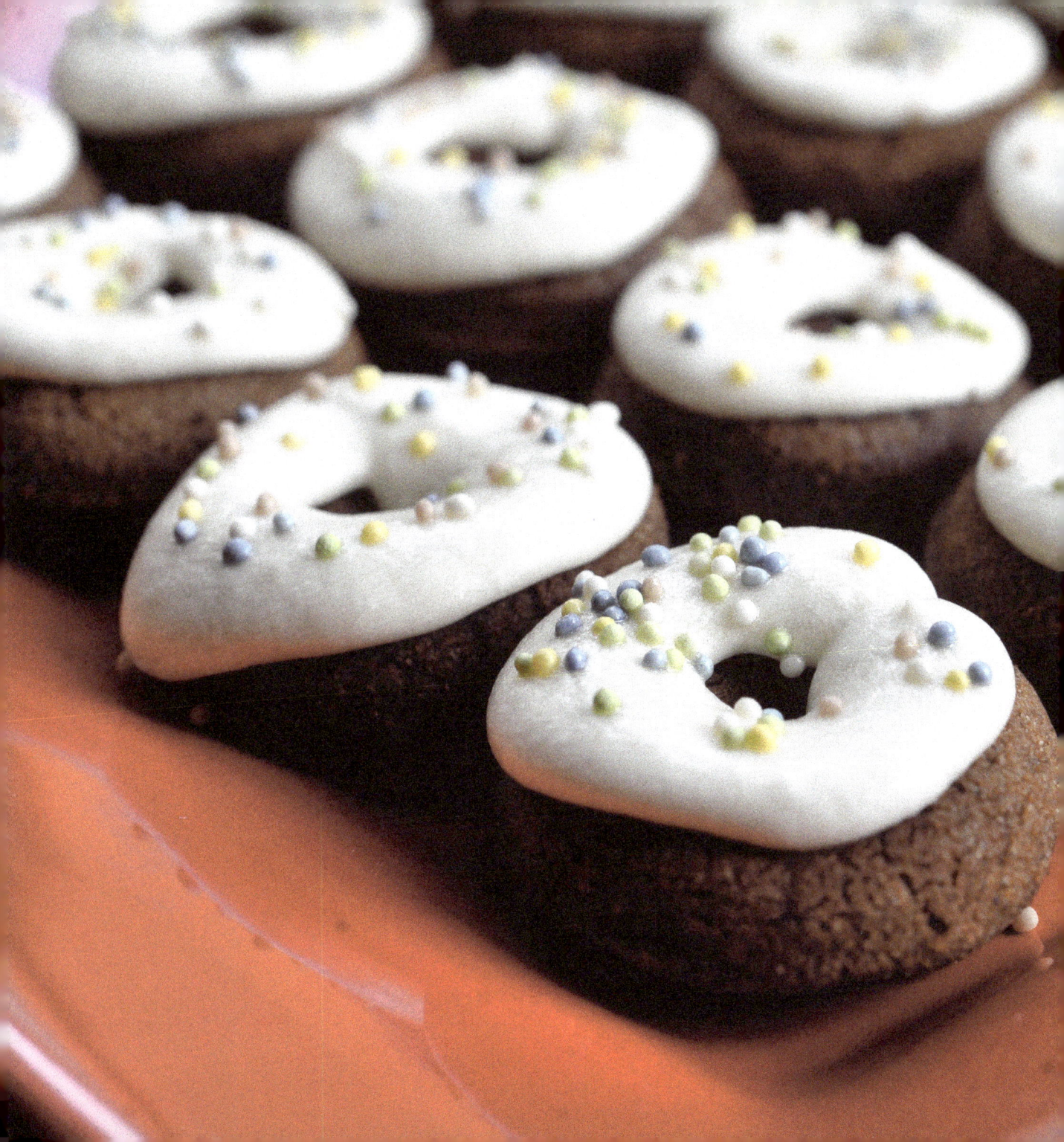

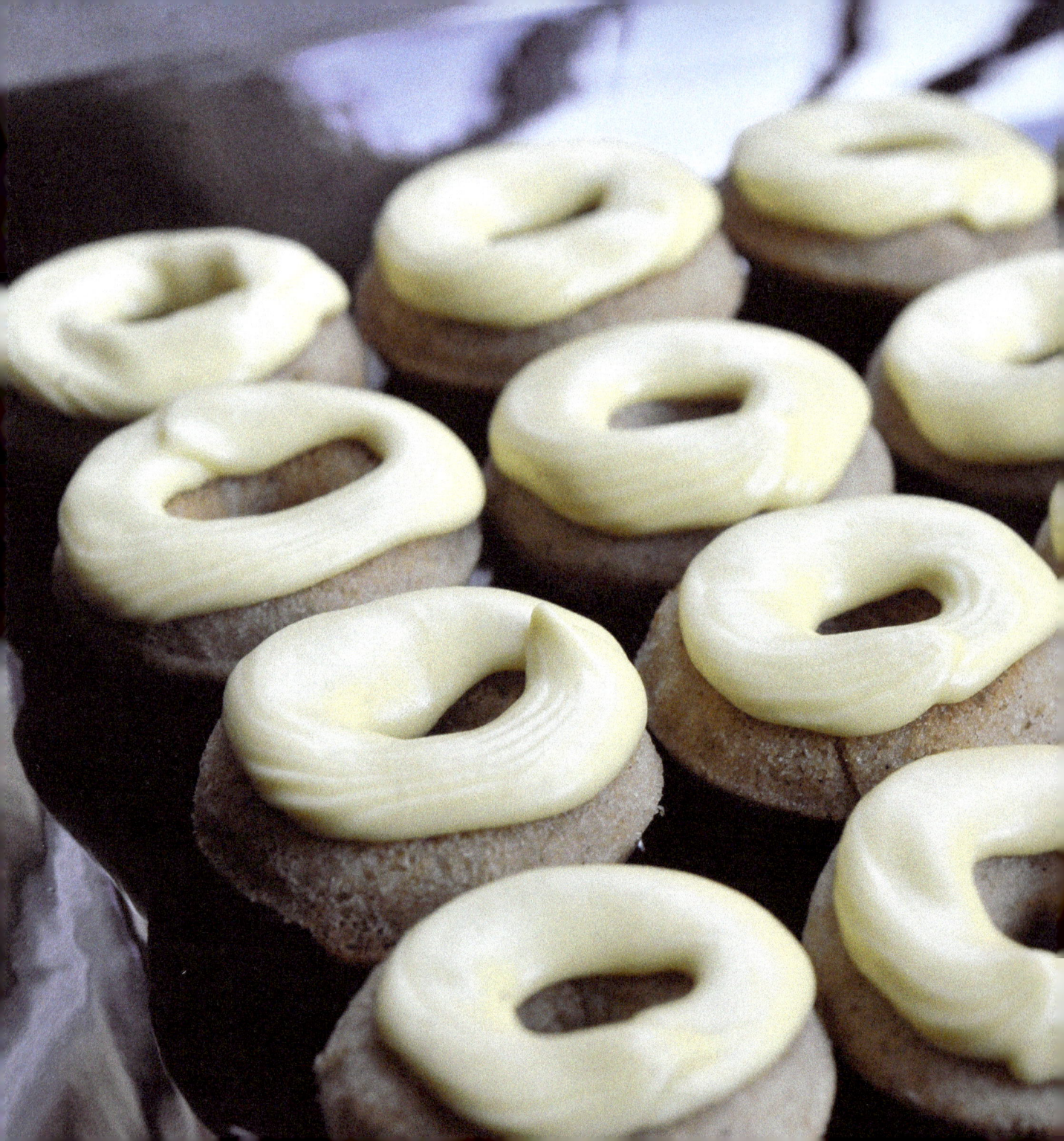

Cake Doughnut with Lemon Icing

Gluten, Dairy, Egg Free
Nut & Soy Free Compatible

Nut Free: Use safe milk.
Soy Free: Use safe butter.

Ingredients:

3 TBSP Dairy Free Butter

1/4 cup Organic Sugar

1 TBSP Potato Starch

1 tsp Baking Powder

Dash of Sea Salt

1/2 cup + 1 TBSP Unsweetened Almond Milk

1 cup White Sorghum Flour

2 tsp Organic Vanilla Extract

Icing:

2 TBSP Dairy Free Butter, room temp.

1 cup Organic Powdered Sugar

Dash of Sea Salt

1/2 tsp Organic Vanilla Extract

1 TBSP Water

1/8 tsp Organic Lemon Extract

Directions:

Review the notes on page 64 before starting.

Using the wire attachment on your mixer, combine the doughnut ingredients on medium speed. Once everything is incorporated, place batter into a decorating bag. This will help ensure accurate placement of the batter.

Cut the tip off of the decorating bag and pipe the batter into your (pre-heated) doughnut maker. I found that 3 minutes in the doughnut maker was a good amount of time.

Allow the doughnuts to cool by "hanging" them on a skewer over a bowl before icing. These have a short shelf life of less than 36 hours, so it's best to serve them fresh.

If you add color to your icing, be careful, as the extra liquid can cause the icing to become runny. Try to plan ahead and make the icing thicker by using less water.

Maple Doughnut with Cinnamon Icing

Gluten, Dairy, Egg Free
Nut & Soy Free Compatible

Nut Free: Use safe milk.
Soy Free: Use safe butter.

This rendition of the doughnut was my favorite to create. It was also well received by the taste tasters.

Ingredients:

3 TBSP Dairy Free Butter

1/4 cup Organic Maple Sugar

1 TBSP Potato Starch

1 tsp Baking Powder

Dash of Sea Salt

1/2 cup Milk, we used Unsweetened Almond Milk

3/4 cup White Sorghum Flour

1 tsp Organic Vanilla Extract

Icing:

2 TBSP Dairy Free Butter, room temp.

1 cups Organic Powdered Sugar (1 standard bag)

Dash of Sea Salt

1/2 tsp Organic Vanilla Extract

1 TBSP Water

1/4 tsp Organic Ground Cinnamon

4 Dashes of Organic Ground Nutmeg

Directions:

Review the notes on page 64 before starting.

Using the wire attachment on your mixer, combine the doughnut ingredients on medium speed. Once everything is incorporated, place batter into a decorating bag. This will help ensure accurate placement of the batter.

Cut the tip off of the decorating bag and pipe the batter into your (pre-heated) doughnut maker. I found that 3 minutes in the doughnut maker was a good amount of time.

Allow the doughnuts to cool by "hanging" them on a skewer over a bowl before icing. These have a short shelf life of less than 36 hours, so it's best to serve them fresh.

If you add color to your icing, be careful, as the extra liquid can cause the icing to become runny. Try to plan ahead and make the icing thicker by using less water.

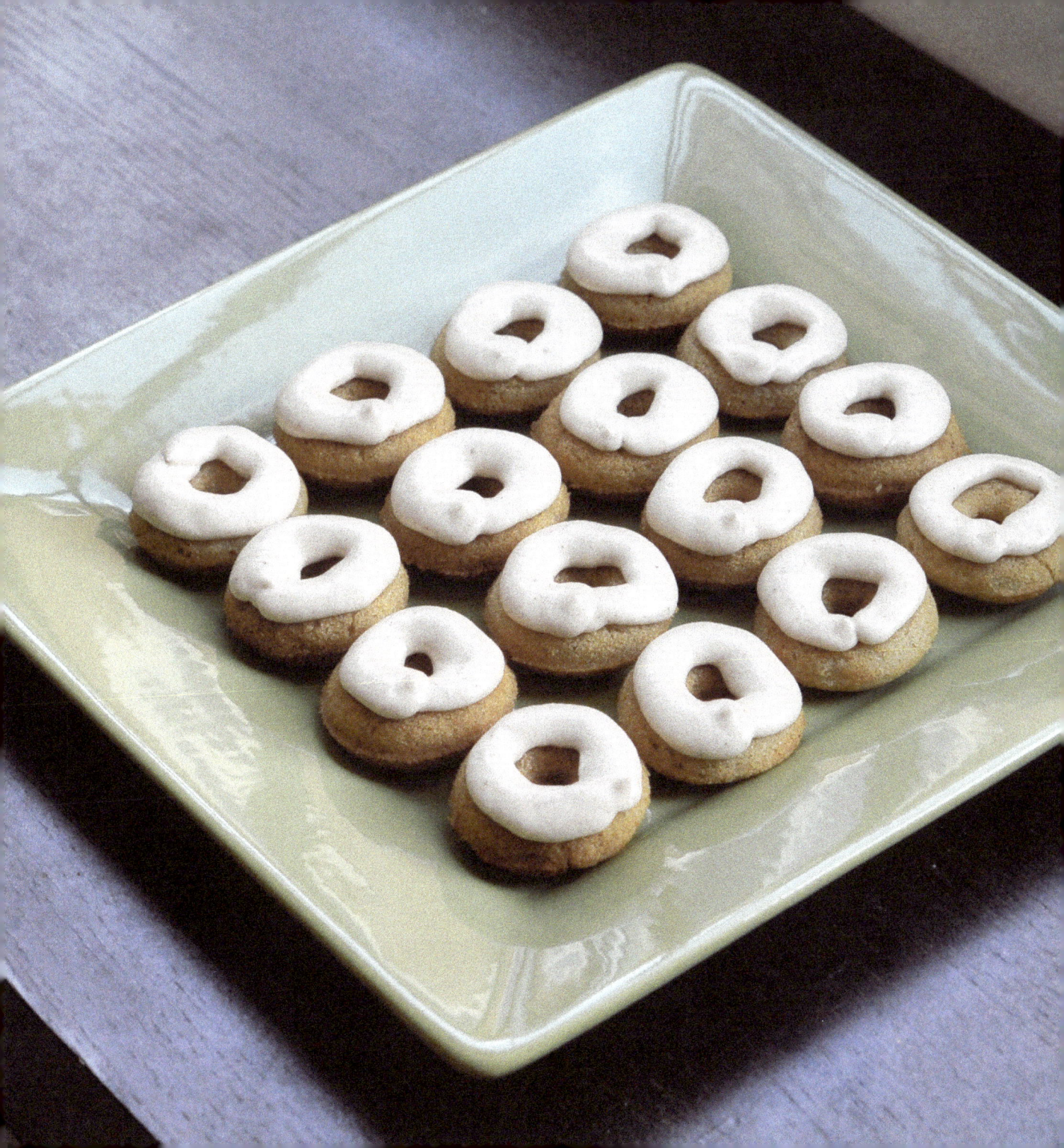

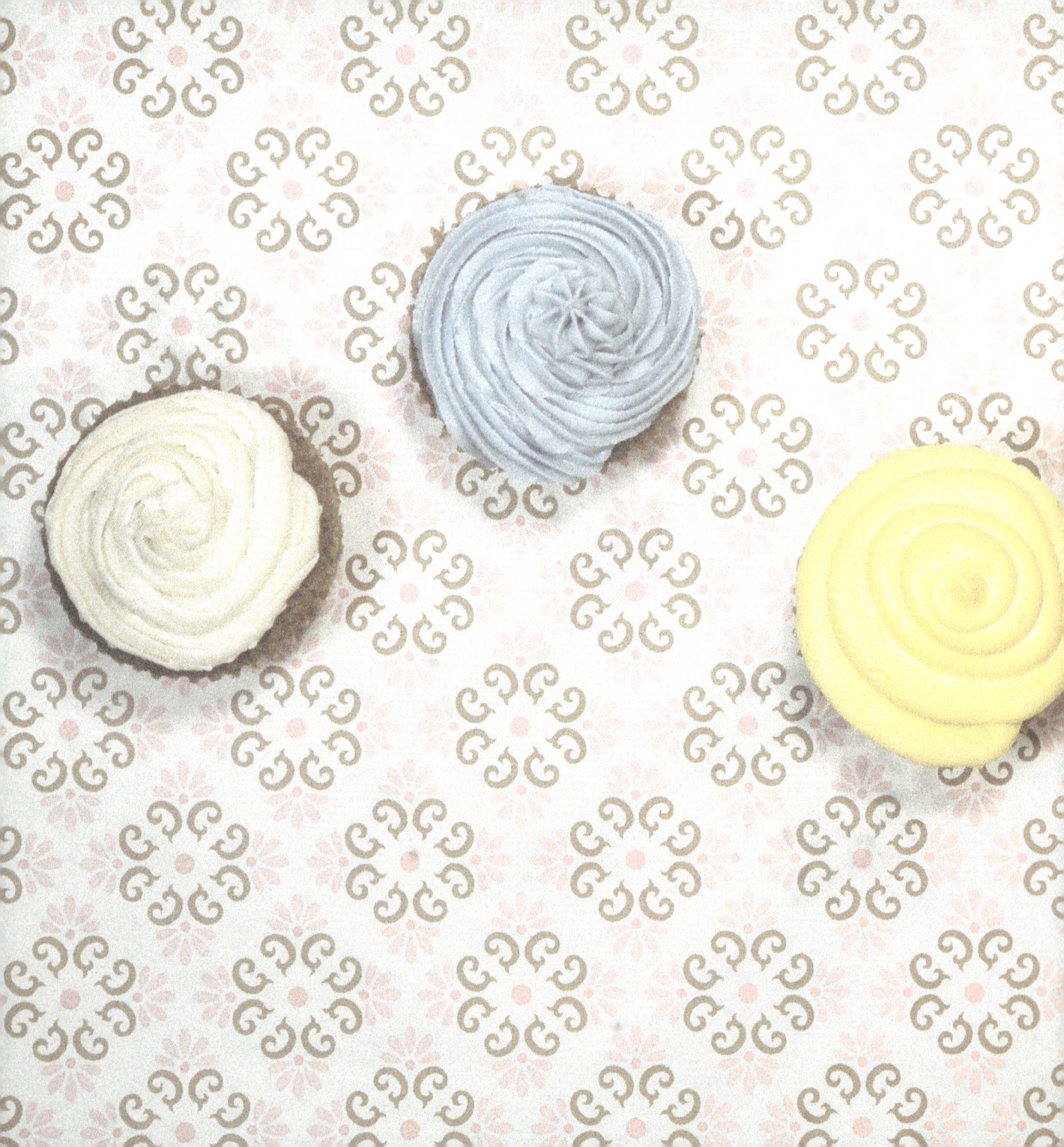

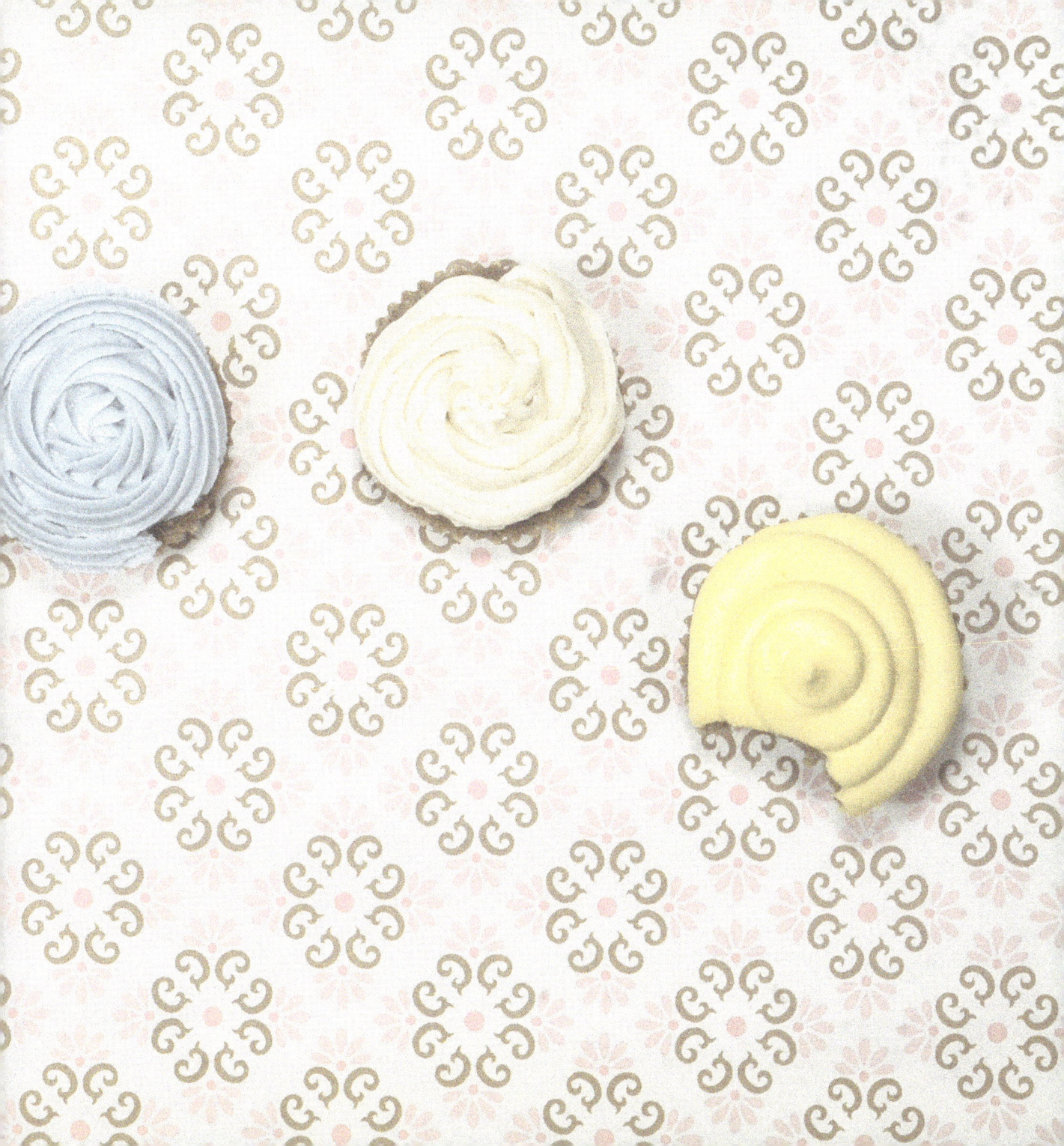

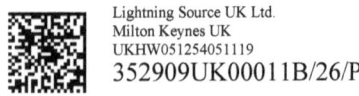